The Future of Orthopaedic Sports Medicine

Brian M. Devitt • Mustafa Karahan
João Espregueira-Mendes
Editors

The Future of Orthopaedic Sports Medicine

What Should We Be Worried About?

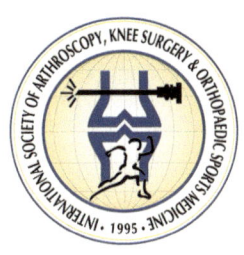

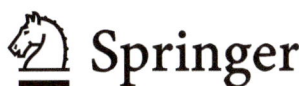

Editors
Brian M. Devitt
OrthoSport Victoria
Melbourne, VIC
Australia

João Espregueira-Mendes
Clínica do Dragão, Espregueira-Mendes
Sports Centre – FIFA Medical Centre of
Excellence, Porto
Braga
Portugal

Mustafa Karahan
Department of Orthopaedics
Acıbadem Mehmet Ali Aydinlar University
Istanbul
Turkey

ISBN 978-3-030-28975-1   ISBN 978-3-030-28976-8   (eBook)
https://doi.org/10.1007/978-3-030-28976-8

This Springer imprint is published by the registered company Springer Nature Switzerland AG
The registered company address is: Gewerbestrasse 11, 6330 Cham, Switzerland

Preface

I used to do my best worrying on a plane. I could worry about all manner of things, some logical, most irrational, but all inconsequential: Would there be enough space in the overhead bin for my bag? Would that screaming child at the gate be sitting next to me? Did I bring my noise cancelling earphones? Would I get off this plane alive?

My propensity to worry in this environment did not reflect my normal disposition and I came to realise that what I was experiencing was a simple case of anticipatory anxiety. I was obviously a little unsettled about relinquishing control of my own destiny and placing it in the hands of a complete stranger in control of an aluminium tube being propelled by a jet engine, high in the air, at vast speeds. What's the big deal?

The reassuring thing for me is that I am not alone in my worries. A quick glance at my fellow passengers on any flight confirms that a large number of them occupy a similar state of discomposure. I try to do my best to avoid eye contact with the worrywarts lest their grimaced faces might betray a fear I haven't yet conceived. Instead, I like to focus on the more serene passengers, most of whom are usually reading a book, probably a form of cognitive therapy to allay their own anxieties. It was on one such occasion, with my mind riddled with angst, that I came across a man reading the book which provided the stimulus for the current manuscript:

What should we be worried about?, edited by John Brockman.

The concept of the book, as proposed by the critically acclaimed author, was to ask leading figures in the world of science to answer a question that inspired unpredictable answers—'*that provoke people into thinking thoughts they normally might not have*'. The result was a compelling book with contributions from approximately 100 authors, who wrote a short essay on a topic of their choice related to the question.

As it happened the man reading the book was my colleague and co-editor of this book, Professor Mustafa Karahan. The flight in question marked the first leg of our travelling fellowship in Asia with a group of ESSKA (European Society of Sports Traumatology, Knee Surgery and Arthroscopy) fellows. Professor Karahan was acting in the role of senior ambassador or godfather, as the position was colloquially known. The poor man hardly got a look in on the book over the next three weeks, as

I stole it away from him on every occasion. Each contribution I read was more thought provoking than the next and provided a catalyst for riveting conversations amongst our group about the future of our own speciality, orthopaedic sports medicine. We decided that we needed to write a book of our own.

Orthopaedic sports medicine as a speciality is diverse. It is composed of a wide array of different specialists, surgeons, physiotherapists, sports physicians and allied health professionals. The exponential growth of this nascent speciality has also been greatly enhanced by the development of strong links with the bioengineering industry and the multitude of technological advancements which this partnership has yielded. As such, and in order to get a true reflection of the '*worries*' or concerns of all the key stakeholders in our speciality, we posed our question not simply to experienced orthopaedic sports surgeons but to all of those involved in our field. To paraphrase an Irish song, we invited '*the young, the old, the brave, and the bold*' to answer the question: The future of orthopaedic sports medicine: What should we be worried about?

The result, as you will read, is a fascinating insight into the worries, fears and anxieties of senior orthopaedic surgeons established in practice, young doctors taking the first fledgling steps in their career, the original pioneers of the field now retired, industry leaders and world renowned scientists, to name but a few. Unlike modern publications which often have a list of co-authors, each piece in this book is written by the author alone. This is based on the premise that what worries a senior physician may not necessarily worry her junior colleague!

In his own words, John Brockman contends that '*the reason why people worry is because we are built to anticipate the future. Nothing can stop us from worrying, but science can teach us how to worry better, and when to stop worrying*'. Although, this may be true, the practice of medicine is not simply about science. To understand human emotions and alleviate anxieties, we must also be able to impart empathy and compassion. So the next time you see that frightened look in your patient's eyes prior to surgery, hold his hand and reassure him. After all, he is about to relinquish control of his own destiny, placing it in the hands of a complete stranger in control of a breathing tube while another masked stranger wields an air saw oscillating at high speeds. What's the big deal?

Melbourne, VLC, Australia   Brian M. Devitt

In memorium: Dr John A Feagin, Jr.

Start by doing what's necessary; then do what's possible; and suddenly you are doing the impossible.

—**Francis of Assisi**

John Feagin was supposed to write this foreword, but sadly he died before completing it. He was one of the forefathers of orthopaedic sports medicine. But, more than that, he was my friend and mentor. I am far from unique in this regard, as this was a role he filled for generations of orthopaedic surgeons throughout the world, many of whom have contributed to this manuscript.

He strongly supported the creation of this book and the question it posed. I shared with him many of the chapters, which he eagerly awaited. He derived great amusement from reading the assortment of worries that tormented his junior colleagues. When I approached him about writing the foreword, I gave him a simple brief. I wanted him to tell us what life was like when he started his career and the speciality of orthopaedic sports medicine was but a twinkle in his eye. So, in his absence, let us reflect on his career through his eyes.

Ironically, for a man whose greatest attribute was perhaps his vision, John's path into medicine came about because of a lack of it. He desperately wanted to become an Air Force pilot like his father. To this end, he attended West Point Military Academy. Unfortunately for John, his visual acuity did not meet the grade required for the Air Force. Disappointed but undeterred, he committed himself to the army. To begin with, his path wasn't clear but while on deployment, as he put it, '*I saw the light. I was going to become a surgeon*' [1].

He treasured above all the privilege of military medicine and caring for the wounded soldier. In this capacity, a thorough knowledge of orthopaedics was crucial. However, even a superior knowledge, at that time, was insufficient in managing soft tissue injuries of the knee, a condition which was highly prevalent amongst military cadets. The shortcomings related to a lack of a thorough understanding of the mechanism of injury, patho-anatomy, diagnosis, classification, and appropriate treatment of these injuries. Through his career, John worked tirelessly to fill this knowledge void.

A problem shared is a problem halved.

In recognising the mammoth nature of this task, he knew this problem was not for solving alone. John sought out fellow surgeons, through the military and beyond, facing the same challenges, and they put their collective minds to the task. The results can be seen in a list of his achievements: founding member of the American Orthopaedic Society for Sports Medicine (AOSSM), member of the International Knee Documentation Committee, co-founder of the Anterior Cruciate Ligament Study Group, co-founder of the Travelling Fellowship programme, esteemed author, and much more. But, to focus on his achievements alone fails to capture the man nor does it do his legacy justice. It was his leadership, unerring positivity, and commitment to lifelong learning that stood him out as a true gentleman and beacon in the field of orthopaedic sports medicine.

His philosophy was always one of inclusion and he loathed elitism. At every opportunity, he welcomed new members and promoted young surgeons, whom he encouraged to think differently and to dispute conventional knowledge. He recognised that as an emerging specialty an insular mindset would be a handbrake to progress, and he steadfastly promoted the cultivation of a relationship with industry to embrace and harness technology.

Such was the peripatetic nature of military life that when John left the army he was left with the permanent affliction of an itchy foot. He travelled widely through his career for work. But, whether it was caring for cowboys or skiers in Jackson Hole, Wyoming, or educating young aspiring surgeons at Duke University, he brought the same vigour and enthusiasm to his tasks. It is also probably why he saw such value in the concept of a travelling fellowship, the establishment of which he ranked as the proudest achievement of his professional career.

The travelling fellowship was created along with his close friends and colleagues, Ejnar Erickson from Sweden and Werner Mueller from Switzerland. It provided a link between the AOSSM and European Society for Sports Traumatology, Knee Surgery and Arthroscopy. Together, they acknowledged that although treatment philosophies often differed between countries, true progress in the field could best be realised by embracing the human side of orthopaedics and sharing openly and honestly not only successful cases but especially failures. Their vision continues to thrive and has made the world of orthopaedic sports medicine a much smaller and better place.

So, what did John think about the future of orthopaedic sports medicine? In a wonderful interview with John Tokish, MD, in 2014, he stated that he *'vastly underestimated the potential of sports medicine. Yet, even now, we are at the tip of the iceberg'* [1]. As I sit and write these words, I can see John's face smiling down at me. I feel his hand gripping my shoulder tightly. I hear his words clearly in my ears, spoken in his soft Texan drawl: *'The best is yet to come, the best is yet to come!'*

Thank you, John, for what you have given us and for what is yet to come!

Melbourne, VLC, Australia											Brian M. Devitt

Reference

1. Tokish JA. Pioneers in orthopaedics. Pioneer—John A Feagin, Jr. 2014. https://www.healio.com/orthopedics/sports-medicine/news/print/orthopedics-today/%7B8299a2f4-67c8-492f-9715-3658840ae903%7D/pioneer-john-a-feagin-jr-md

Contents

How Long Is a Piece of String?

Joanna M. Stephen

Opinions are very prevalent in the field of orthopaedics. Indeed, a significant proportion of current clinical interventions are conducted on the basis of these opinions. However, all too often, these opinions lack robust scientific evidence that should arguably be in place to support their application. Surely, we should be better equipped by now to challenge such dogma. Sports medicine is an active research field with an abundance of publications in a rapidly growing number of journals. It is an attractive field that engages many young, talented researchers. Yet, despite this, opinions remain more common than science. One reason for this, and my primary worry for moving the profession forward, is the clear lack of robust, objective measurement techniques in sports medicine. I strongly believe that basic science holds the fundamental foundation that should enable us to advance the field and promote successful outcomes in patients but that the need for this is not widely appreciated.

Considering this, I am taken back to a UK documentary where the narrator tried to answer the common English phrase, 'how long is a piece of string?' This is a humorous phrase, typically stated in response to a question for which there is no definitive answer. The narrator is followed taking a length of string to a series of mathematicians and physicists and asking whether they can determine how long it is. This quickly becomes more complicated than first appears. The exact definition of what has to be measured must be agreed. In the case of the string, is the length measured along its central axis or along one edge? Where exactly are the ends of the string? Should the string be lying flat or hanging up? How straight does the string need to be during measurement? Each of these variables will clearly influence the end measurement and is therefore given due consideration by the scientists. Secondly, they must select an outcome tool to perform the measurement. 'Eyeballing' with a ruler is the obvious first option, but significant errors and variables are

J. M. Stephen (✉)
Fortius Clinic, London, UK

Department of Mechanical Engineering, Imperial College London, London, UK
e-mail: j.stephen10@imperial.ac.uk

© ISAKOS 2020   1
B. M. Devitt et al. (eds.), *The Future of Orthopaedic Sports Medicine*,
https://doi.org/10.1007/978-3-030-28976-8_1

identified. After much deliberation and a few button presses on a laser tracker, the three-dimensional positions of the ends of string are determined and its length calculated. The method is simpler, faster and with significantly less error than the manual measurement. It made me think, such measures could be tremendously useful in orthopaedics. So I am left to wonder, why do we not apply such technology to orthopaedic measures? This could remove human error and ensure consistency of objective measures across studies all over the world.

In orthopaedic sports medicine, we measure physical quantities on a daily basis: the laxity in a joint, the position of a tunnel for soft tissue reconstruction, the alignment of a bone or joint, etc. Most commonly, in clinical practice, these are quantified with 'eyeballing' or subjective feel. However, as with the string, each of these measures will be affected by variables such as weight-bearing status, the axes to which the joint or bones are aligned and the plane (or planes) in which, the measurements are taken. If only it could be as simple as measuring that piece of string—two clicks and the answer appears. But why can it not be? Similar to the laser and string, in the digital era, tools are widely available in the world that are capable of making measurements in orthopaedics more robust; repeatable and, all the while, simpler, cheaper and faster. Why if these tools are available are they not used? How do we encourage the development of a more multi-disciplinary approach to research?

In an era striving for precision medicine, we must successfully harness modern technology if we are to advance our understanding of musculoskeletal pathology. It appears the case that we need better research using reliable measurement devices and protocols. The development of standardised, repeatable and valid objective measurements must be a priority, particularly, if we are to compare data from across the world and generate the large databases necessary to drive sports medicine forwards. There is a clear need to reform the culture that rewards the quantity of publications as a measure of ability, with a greater focus instead on quality and validity of studies. The fostering of an open and collaborative approach to research, actively seeking and welcoming scientists from other fields to work alongside us and contribute their unique knowledge and skills to improve what we do. The realisation of funding councils that the development of objective measurements is a crucial and a very worthwhile long-term investment. This is all possible, and some of it is already taking place. Therefore, my greatest concern, I believe, also represents the greatest challenge and opportunity in sports medicine. What a great era to be a scientist.

Finally, how long was that piece of string? Well, it depends; how long do we need it to be?

Mustafa Karahan

Our job requires constant decision making, followed by application of these decisions into practice. It is the core of our profession. We select a logical choice from the available options day in, day out, constantly, be it selecting the optimal treatment for a degenerative meniscal tear in a middle-aged individual or a first-time shoulder dislocator in an adolescent athlete.

Logic is concerned with the principles of correct reasoning. There are a number of categories of logic that exist. Formal logic is the classical system of determining the validity or invalidity of a conclusion deduced from two or more statements. Informal logic refers to the principles of logic outside of a formal setting. It is commonly regarded as an alternative to formal logic and usually called inductive logic. Reasoning based on informal/inductive logic reaches a conclusion that extrapolates from, amplifies, or generalizes the evidence. Inductive reasoning is prone to fallacies, which is commonly seen in daily life and clinical practice. The following are some of the common examples of inductive logic that we may encounter in our clinics:

He is not a good surgeon, because he has no publications

- **Ad Hominem**: Latin for "against the person." Attacking a person based on irrelevant issues.

It can't be true, I have never seen a case like this.

- **Argument from Ignorance**: Claiming something cannot be true simply because one has never experienced it.

Platelet Rich Plasma is the choice, because it has become very popular recently.

M. Karahan (✉)
Department of Orthopaedics, Acıbadem Mehmet Ali Aydınlar University, Istanbul, Turkey

© ISAKOS 2020
B. M. Devitt et al. (eds.), *The Future of Orthopaedic Sports Medicine*,
https://doi.org/10.1007/978-3-030-28976-8_2

- **Bandwagon Appeal**: Popularity does not necessarily mean something is better, safer, or truer than something else.

  I tenotomize the biceps in all rotator cuff rupture cases. I believe I am right since no one cannot prove I am wrong.

- **Begging the Question**: If someone is not wrong, then that someone must, by definition be right but not necessarily the narrator.

  Dr. Devitt is a great surgeon, because he is very particular during surgery.

- **Circular Reasoning**: The second sentence does not necessarily actually explain why Dr. Devitt is so great.

  Prof. Smith is a kind person, I should apply for a fellowship in his clinic.

- **Emotional Appeal**: It is illogical to base an argument primarily or solely on emotional grounds.

  Arthroscopic debridement works in the shoulder, so it must work in the knee.

- **False Analogy**: Comparison between two things that are not really similar.

  You should choose either arthroscopic debridement or unicompartmental arthroplasty in medial compartment knee osteoarthritis.

- **False Dilemma**: A false dilemma involves the insistence on only two alternatives when there may be others.

  I quit scoping shoulders, it always bleeds.

- **Hasty Generalization**: Making an inductive leap on the basis of too little evidence.

  My patient developed reflex sympathetic dystrophy (RSD) after arthroscopic meniscectomy. Loss of meniscus causes RSD.

- **Post Hoc Fallacy**: The fallacy maintains that because event B happened after event A, and A must have caused B. This is not necessarily true; it can be true, but the cause and effect must be *proven*, not merely assumed.

  If you surgically stabilize a first time shoulder dislocation, you may damage the cartilage, cause infection and cause severe secondary osteoarthritis.

- **Slippery Slope**: This involves extending a chain of logic beyond the point at which it is reasonably acceptable.

Because they are extremely difficult, I am the only one in the region that takes on revision ACL cases.

• **Straw Man**: The statement invites others to reject a person or a group based on an exaggerated or distorted characterization.

The logical limitation of evidence-based medicine is that clinical decisions should be based exclusively on the so-called "best evidence," without the use of inductive reasoning. However, since it is not always possible to consider all possible factors while answering a clinical question, medical decision making will always require inductive reasoning. While doing so, one should not fall into the persuasiveness of the easy and common thinking, which will lead us to stray us away from the truth.

Fiachra Rowan

I'm lucky to live and work in a coastal city at the edge of the Atlantic Ocean. Weekends are typically spent near the water. Frequently, however, my children and I fill our arms with washed up plastic waste as we turn for home. I used to despair at how other humans could pollute the world in this way, but then I realised I'm no better. I consider myself environmentally aware: I rarely buy bottled water; I always refuse the plastic lid for my coffee and I never use plastic bags. But the moment I open my single-use, pre-packed gown and gloves in the operating room, I'm no better than the rest. A routine medial patellofemoral ligament reconstruction, anterior cruciate ligament reconstruction or even chondral repair fills at least three refuse sacks. Yes, some will be recycled, but somewhere between 20% and 70% of joint replacement waste is hazardous and will go for incineration or landfill and eventually enter the food chain [1, 2].

When I compare the implant to applicator and packaging weight ratio between arthroscopic and arthroplasty knee surgery, the more invasive joint replacement generates less. Of course, this is down to the mass of metal alloys versus plastics, but our advances in surgery have had an environmental impact. Improvements in sterilisation for longevity and sterility have resulted in layers of plastics that are lightweight but voluminous. The tactile feedback and performance of market leading interference screws or meniscal repair systems have certainly revolutionised knee surgery and patient outcomes, but it is now time to return to the design table. A hip arthroscopy may generate a modest 9 kg of waste compared with 15 kg for a TKA, but multiple refuse bags are produced, of which only 7% may be recyclable [2, 3]. We need to reduce or re-use materials, not rely on recycling.

Single-use supporters would highlight the excesses of decontamination, sterilisation and repackaging, but this can be overcome by using renewable energy,

F. Rowan (✉)
Department of Trauma and Orthopaedic Surgery, University Hospital Waterford,
Waterford, Ireland
e-mail: fr@fiachrarowan.com

© ISAKOS 2020   7
B. M. Devitt et al. (eds.), *The Future of Orthopaedic Sports Medicine*,
https://doi.org/10.1007/978-3-030-28976-8_3

recaptured water systems and recycled materials. Improvements in recycling practices are commendable, but the recycling industry is an industry and the industry consumes energy and produces waste. The plastic production industry itself accounts for 8% of annual world oil and gas expenditure. We should be reducing our plastic use or even seeking to re-use some materials. We can no longer expect other countries to launder our recycling. Compostable and biodegradable "plastics" do not provide the answer either. Such materials are frequently produced from plants, a resource that is increasingly compromised by global climate change and Western consumption.

Surgical pollution is what I worry about. Sure, I worry about my surgical performance and how my patients do under my care, but I'm a surgical polluter and I worry that little is being done about it. The European Union's recent Medical Devices Regulation (2017) tightens legislation on hazardous material use in manufacturing, but it seems that an opportunity to improve surgical packaging and single-use materials has been missed for the environment [4]. We need to remember that the planet is a patient under all our care.

References

1. Stall NM, Kagoma YK, Bondy JN, Naudie D. Surgical waste audit of 5 total knee arthroplasties. Can J Surg. 2013;56(2):97–102.
2. Lee RJ, Mears SC. Reducing and recycling in joint Arthroplasty. J Arthroplast. 2012;27(10):1757–60.
3. de SAD, Stephens K, Kuang M, Simunovic N, Karlsson J, Ayeni OR. The direct environmental impact of hip arthroscopy for femoroacetabular impingement: a surgical waste audit of five cases. J Hip Preserv Surg. 2016;3(2):132–7.
4. EUR-Lex—32017R0745–EN—EUR-Lex. https://eur-lex.europa.eu/legal-content/EN/TXT/?uri=CELEX:32017R0745.

Are We Losing Our Profession Through the Loss of Leadership?

Dean C. Taylor

I do my best not to worry. As my mentor Jim Urbaniak is fond of saying, "Worry is irrational concern." Although not worried, I am deeply concerned about the future of Sports Medicine. I am concerned that many physicians do not accept their responsibility to be ethical leaders in our profession. I am concerned that without a commitment to ethical leadership, we are becoming technicians, losing the capacity to provide humanitarian care, and abdicating to administrators our responsibility to lead.

Healthcare leadership is the ability to influence others for the benefit of patients and patient populations. The core principle that differentiates healthcare leadership from leadership in other fields is patient-centeredness (Fig. 4.1 [1]). The overlapping and complementary competencies that effective healthcare leaders possess include emotional intelligence, critical thinking, teamwork, integrity, and selfless service.

Effective leadership in healthcare is essential for Sports Medicine physicians. Sports Medicine is complex and becoming more so. No longer can the omnipotent physician "leader" exist in this complex world. Instead, the complexity dictates a team approach. Physicians through experience and education are logical leaders for these teams; however, we often shirk our leadership responsibility, or exhibit ineffective or abhorrent leadership behavior. With very little thought, I am sure you can think of a time you or one of your colleagues avoided contributing to a hospital initiative that administrators mismanaged. Or maybe there was a time where you acted disrespectfully toward a team member and that action disrupted the team chemistry and morale. On reflection, you probably realize that it may have taken care of the issue in that moment, but in the long term, your patients were negatively affected by the breakdown in trust and teamwork that such behavior creates.

D. C. Taylor (✉)
Duke University, Durham, NC, USA
e-mail: dean.taylor@duke.edu

© ISAKOS 2020 9
B. M. Devitt et al. (eds.), *The Future of Orthopaedic Sports Medicine*,
https://doi.org/10.1007/978-3-030-28976-8_4

Fig. 4.1 Duke healthcare
leadership model [1]

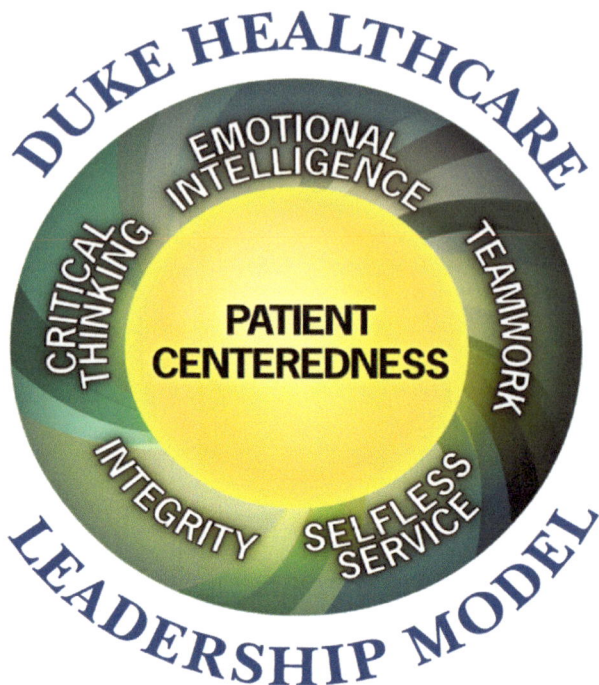

I am concerned that instead of intentionally emphasizing effective, ethical leadership competencies, we are modeling behavior that is more movivated by self-interest. Such behavior is frequently unintentional. It is often the result of low self-awareness and poor self-management, a reflection of inadequate emotional intelligence, and a lack of the critical thinking necessary to appreciate bias.

For example, consider the field of Orthobiologics. Skilled researchers have identified exciting agents (PRP, stem cells, etc.) that hold tremendous therapeutic promise. Some are aggressively marketing these investigational orthobiologic therapies and profiting handsomely, without the rigorous research that should accompany investigational treatments. Although this behavior is not widespread, it is growing, and those not involved, are not actively questioning it. Our professional organizations are not questioning this behavior either but are allowing educational offerings and promotions of new therapies that are biased by industry money and underemphasized conflicts of interest (think about the time spent on the second "Disclosure" slide of every talk at professional meetings). Ultimately, will our lack of responsive leadership contribute to a rising public perception of Sports Medicine as a specialty of hucksters and charlatans, out for profit with little care for the patient? Although this damning perception may not reflect the reality of physicians trying to help patients with the latest treatments they believe in, perception is reality, and perceptions lead to consequences. The reality is that those consequences are greater regulation and loss of professional autonomy due to our inability to effectively lead our profession.

How do we address my concerns? Individually, each of us must accept responsibility to be effective, ethical leaders. We have to show up—the first rule of leadership—and we have to continually learn to be better leaders, just as we continually learn to be technically better surgeons.

Organizationally, ISAKOS and all professional entities must work diligently to create cultures that are unwaveringly committed to leadership education and support ethical leadership competencies. We need to intentionally emphasize, just as we emphasize surgical technique education, educational offerings on leadership competencies such as teamwork and emotional intelligence, which will lead to better patient care. We need to create patient-centered cultures that promote selfless service and are steadfast in upholding integrity.

We all need to be effective, ethical Sports Medicine leaders. If we do not, then we will become technicians answering to managers, and my greatest concern will be realized—there will no longer exist a Sports Medicine profession to lead.

Reference

1. Hargett CW, Doty JP, Hauck JN, Webb AM, Cook SH, Tsipis NE, et al. Developing a model for effective leadership in healthcare: a concept mapping approach. J Healthc Leadersh. 2017;9:69–78.

BIG DATA: Revolution or Complication?

5

Etienne Cavaignac

When I got the email from the ISAKOS inviting me to contribute a chapter for this book, the first thing that came to mind was the French cartoon hero Asterix: 'The Gauls have only one fear: that the sky may fall on their heads tomorrow'. Although I do not fear the sky falling, I do worry about how Big Data will impact Orthopaedic Sports Medicine; big data refers to large volumes of data and the vast analysis possibilities.

Modern communication, storage and computing technologies have allowed the data analytics field to take a quantum leap forward. It is now possible to analyse data on a population level, not only in a group of subjects. This change in paradigm is called big data analysis. In this chapter, I will focus only on the analysis of large volumes of data, not on ethical problems or consequences related to analysing and predicting behaviours.

First, the explosion in the volume of available data brings up a question of relevance: Which data is relevant to us as clinicians? One of my previous supervisors regularly explained to us that we could make slices with a precision of one-tenth of a millimetre in aeronautics, but that this level of precision is not useful in masonry. The end goal of the analysis must be at the forefront, not the method used. The number of outcome measures in a study is less important than the quality of these outcomes. However, there is no universal definition of quality outcome—it all depends on what we want to study. Relevance is key, but its definition varies.

What do we need to know for sports medicine? In my opinion, the only relevant outcome is patient satisfaction. Functional scores are only a futile attempt at standardisation. Other objective outcomes do not reflect on the success of the treatment either. Patient satisfaction is multifactorial. It captures the patient's wishes, understanding of the treatment pathway, expected outcome and the actual outcome (not an exhaustive list). Because it is multifactorial, satisfaction is a comprehensive

E. Cavaignac (✉)
Department of Orthopaedic Surgery, Hopital Pierre Paul Riquet, CHU Toulouse, Toulouse, France

© ISAKOS 2020
B. M. Devitt et al. (eds.), *The Future of Orthopaedic Sports Medicine*,
https://doi.org/10.1007/978-3-030-28976-8_5

assessment. Unfortunately, it is harder to normalise the analysis of satisfaction on a population scale. Nevertheless, a satisfied patient means that the medical team has addressed all the prerequisites for optimal patient care.

Second, we must ask whether all the available collected data should be analysed. A study should be conducted to prove or disprove a hypothesis using a set of outcome measures. Collecting all sorts of data and then determining which variables have a p-value <0.05 misses the point. Early in my career as a clinical scientist, I went to see a young resident in medical statistics for help with my analysis. After a few days, he called me to say the most significant finding was that the patients who were the oldest at the time of enrolment were the most likely to have died at the last follow-up!! Statistically unanswerable but not very relevant. Statistical analysis is a means to an end, not an end in itself. It is used to prove or disprove a hypothesis by factoring in the possibility that the result was obtained by chance.

Big data is being pitched to us as a way to better understand observed phenomena by extensively analysing large data sets. However, the more we analyse a series of cases, the higher the probability that the result will be achieved by chance. Because big data allows us to work with larger databases, it is easy to get caught up in all the findings generated by the analysis. The aim of the analysis must be at the forefront during each step of the research. To obtain a valid answer, we must ask an appropriate research question. While technologies change, our research methodology must continue to be rigorous. Having more data is not as critical as having relevant data.

The Influence of Industry

Peter T. Myers

In my practice, I repair many torn menisci and have been doing so for 30 years. I use a suture shuttle system that I purchased in the early 1990s and continue to use. Trainees, fellows and visiting surgeons who see me use this simple system all want to know how they can get hold of one. They cannot—and this concerns me—the company that made it is long since gone and I think I have the last remaining needles on the planet. This is a reusable system, sterilisable and sturdy. We have had a few replacements made by instrument makers, but they are not as good as the originals. I have asked reputable orthopaedic companies to make it and the simple response is, 'if it is not single use only, then we are not interested'. The cost to produce this system is less than the cost of two single-use all-inside devices; thus, the reluctance of the industry to produce it even though it is easier to use, more accurate, more versatile and more successful than the more profitable all-inside devices. This concerns me, not because of the greediness of the industry but because of cost and patient outcomes.

How much of our acquisition of new knowledge is industry directed? There are industry-sponsored (partly or completely) textbooks, journals, research projects, research fellowships, meetings, lectures, visiting experts, observation programs and others. As surgeons, we are grateful for the industry support for our meetings and other involvements. Indeed, this book is only possible because of ISAKOS, which has some industry support. This concerns me, as it is becoming more difficult to have meaningful debate and learned discussion without an industry bias.

New technology—encompassing techniques, instruments, devices, implants or occasionally a truly new technology—is rarely introduced to the orthopaedic community by learned societies, associations or at unbiased meetings. More commonly, a 'technology' is developed, a use found for it and then a rationale for this use developed and promoted by a surgeon who is loyal to the particular company and put

P. T. Myers (✉)
Brisbae Orthopaedic and Sports Medicine Centre, Brisbane, QLD, Australia
e-mail: p.myers@bosmc.com.au

© ISAKOS 2020
B. M. Devitt et al. (eds.), *The Future of Orthopaedic Sports Medicine*,
https://doi.org/10.1007/978-3-030-28976-8_6

forward as a 'key opinion leader'. The new item is commonly promoted and used in patients long before there is evidence that it is better than what was used previously. New techniques are often introduced on flimsy scientific grounds or only to gain a market share of an otherwise successful procedure. It takes many years of usage and studies to determine whether or not the new technique is truly better. This concerns me, not because of the aggressive nature of the industry but because of the patients who will suffer as a result of the introduction into the market of poorly performing 'new' technologies.

Along with these introductions, there is also a sometimes not so subtle denigration of the pre-existing techniques. This can take the form of implied (or actual) poor results, high complications, excessive cost or technical difficulty, and the assumption is that the new technique will therefore be better. Many established techniques have been forgotten in the race to do the latest usually highly promoted new procedure. The new techniques frequently involve single-use or disposable instruments, a major cost to the healthcare systems but a major boost to industry income with no proven improvement in patient outcomes.

The introduction of computer-driven technology into surgery has taken many forms beginning with computer navigation in its many forms, image-derived instrumentation and robotics. What has driven this? Was there a clinical need? Have our surgical outcomes been so poor as to create a necessity for improved systems? Of course not. However, it is promoted as 'cutting edge', 'patient specific' and is easily assumed by many to be better. The cost of these systems is borne by the hospitals, insurance and health systems and not by the orthopaedic industry, which saves inordinately on the cost of the instrumentation otherwise needed for the surgery. This massive cost shift is to no benefit unless there are significant improvements in patient outcomes. This concerns me because ultimately such cost increases without clinical benefit are not sustainable in healthcare funding.

This is not to say that innovations are not welcome. Indeed, we have seen amazing advances that have benefited patients, and many of these would not have been possible without innovation and industry support. We must take responsibility for the welfare of our patients and not take on new technology simply for the sake of it. Be wary of heavily promoted techniques without good clinical justification and results.

7

Are We Stifling Innovation?

Laurence D. Higgins

> *So much of what we call management consists in making it difficult for people to work.*
>
> —Peter Drucker

The aggregation of power among healthcare systems, covertly cradled under the mantra of improving efficiency, increasing access and enhancing value (bending the so-called 'cost curve'), embodies an existential threat to both creation and adoption of disruptive and cost-effective technologies. This disruption in innovation will ultimately interfere with doing more of the right things rather than doing the wrong things more effectively. The seismic shift in hospital-based employment models for physicians restricts physician participation in competitive ventures, actively disincentivizes collaboration, dampens free trade and directly inhibits innovation. In addition, group purchasing organizations (GPOs) further degrade innovation by restricting free trade and creating artificial barriers to market entry. Their unique congressional exemption to anti-kickback statutes allows manufacturers to provide GPOs with 'administrative fees' (frequently characterized as kickbacks by opponents) designed to block competitive products. We believe that the dramatic cost reductions necessary to transition to more effectively deliver care can only germinate and flourish in an environment conducive to innovation that focuses on outcomes, questions the status quo, embraces teamwork, is inspiring and welcomes experimentation.

The transition to an 'employed' model of healthcare, in and of itself, does not necessarily preclude an innovative environment. What is clear is that the rate of increase in the number of non-physician healthcare administrators is greater than

L. D. Higgins (✉)
Arthrex Inc., Naples, FL, USA
e-mail: Larry.Higgins@Arthrex.com

© ISAKOS 2020   17
B. M. Devitt et al. (eds.), *The Future of Orthopaedic Sports Medicine*,
https://doi.org/10.1007/978-3-030-28976-8_7

the increase in the number of physicians over the last 35 years (3200% administrator growth versus 150% physician growth), which has limited physician opportunities to participate in management and to innovate and optimize healthcare delivery. Hospital consolidation recorded a record 115 transactions in 2017 (with over 30 valued at greater than 1 billion in revenue) and is trending to a 15% year-over-year increase in 2018. Consequently, the growth of large healthcare networks, many with market power over insurers and referring physicians has resulted in a dramatic shift towards a direct physician employment model. Private or group practice models decreased an astonishing 17% from 48% to 31% in the last 5 years and new orthopaedic surgeon graduates became employees of a hospital or health network 14% of the time in 2002 versus 41% of the time in 2012. Such direct employment models often significantly limit or completely capture consulting or royalty-bearing opportunities, further crippling innovation. Annual physician surveys show growing dissatisfaction with bureaucracy and the tenor of the hospital–physician relationships with nearly 50% more physicians describing the relationship between hospitals and physicians as negative. Such environments either preclude or disincentivize both innovation and value creation and may promote apathy and maintenance of the status quo, which is ultimately detrimental for patient care.

While hospital system consolidation and physician employment have been shown to enhance bargaining power of the health system due to size and reduced competition, a perhaps larger threat to innovation is the power and protection that GPOs enjoy in the current marketplace. Vizient, the largest GPO, controls up to 30% of all medical supply expenditures and in aggregate, the four largest GPOs together represent 90% of all medical supply spend. While aggregating hospital spend would certainly lower expenditures if the process was competitive, the current structure of GPOs borders on anti-competitive and, as such, stifles innovation. Briefly, GPOs are exempt from anti-kickback legislation and universally charge medical supply companies an 'administrative fee' that is simply passed onto the consumer and furthermore seek and charge a 'premium' fee for sole source relationships that restrict choice, raise cost, limit competition and prevent small companies with innovative products from competing in the market. This artificial restriction in the supply chain has led to drug and supply shortages (sterile saline was sole sourced in many cases from Baxter Corporation in Puerto Rico, which suffered catastrophic damage from Hurricane Maria), which can negatively impact patient care. A recent analysis from Johns Hopkins exposed anti-innovative behaviour from GPOs that prevented a new pulse oximeter from Masimo from entering the market, as Tyco International had paid for market exclusivity from GPOs in the form of premium administrative fees.

Innovation should be at the core of our strategy to control healthcare costs along with process improvements and decreasing variability. We must vigorously evaluate our environment to ensure that we have aligned our structure and incentives to promote a free market dedicated to ensuring we are doing more of the right things. Ultimately, we have a responsibility to shift the focus back to creating an environment in which success is measured by the value we provide to patients.

Don't Get Dragged into the Gloom: Keep the Flame!

8

Niek Van Dijk

As orthopods, we strive for our patients' welfare. But what about our own? We can't serve our patients, if we are struggling ourselves. In the Journal of ISAKOS (jISA-KOS), I have addressed the problem [1]. The figures are alarming:

- surgeons drink, more than ordinary people (we have 10% more "heavy drinkers") [2, 3].
- surgeons burn-out, in alarming numbers (50%, according to a current report) [4]
- surgeons divorce, more than ordinary people (15% more) [5, 6]
- older surgeons have more health problems, including depression (50% of surgeons over 50) [7]
- surgeons ponder suicide, more than ordinary people [4, 8]
- surgeons consider their work-place "unhealthy," more than other professions [8]

It varies between cultures, as you might expect. Chinese doctors worry about under-payment (with 45% ready to quit) [9]. In USA, they worry about litigation (42% have been sued for malpractice) [10]. It is slightly worse in private practice than in academics (burnout at 43% versus 38%, depression at 33% versus 28%, suicidal-moods at 7% versus 4%, and similarly for career-satisfaction) [8]. Overall, it doesn't look too good [11].

But what is the reason? It's clear that we surgeons work long hours and feel we're always "on duty." In the nineteenth century, everybody worked longer hours under worse conditions. But they just "got on with it" because they had no choice. Modern scholars, entrepreneurs, and the self-employed also work long hours, but they don't take to drink or have breakdowns, as we do.

It's also clear that our work and status have been changing. In my early career, I spent 6% of my time on administration, and surgeons were treated like Gods,

N. Van Dijk (✉)
Department of Orthopaedic, University of Amsterdam, Amsterdam, The Netherlands
e-mail: c.n.vandijk@amc.uva.nl

© ISAKOS 2020
B. M. Devitt et al. (eds.), *The Future of Orthopaedic Sports Medicine*,
https://doi.org/10.1007/978-3-030-28976-8_8

effectively immune from criticism. The average surgeon now spends 44% on "admin" and is increasingly regarded as a soft target.

But these aren't the real problems. We need to grasp that our work is hard, and in a particular way. Most of us encounter disease and decay, and we deal with traffic accidents, with industrial injuries, and the random violence of modern life. In this respect, we're like the military, who routinely deal with life and death. This places a profound burden upon us.

We can learn from the military, and their hard-earned wisdom. Lord Moran argued that resilience, toughness, or endurance is a finite resource like a bank-balance. Everybody starts with some capital, but this can be exhausted, by a single withdrawal, or the daily drip–drip of a difficult life. When the balance drifts into red, there'll be symptoms we can diagnose and act before it's too late. But If we miss the signs, there'll be collapse.

"It is the tough ones you need to watch, the ones who never show the strain, who always keep a calm face. They are the ones you find in middle-age, sitting behind their desks, with the tears pouring down their faces" [12].

In short, we're asking too much of ourselves. Our work is draining, and there's too much of it. Too little is being done to monitor us, and too much to satisfy the bureaucrats. We need to watch our colleagues, and if they're close to failing, we need to get them out, and into rest-and-recreation [13]. Sport is the best form of recreation, as the military also understand. If we do this in time, we can save them. Otherwise, they will fail. They'll turn to drink or drugs, or they'll turn against themselves.

There are other things we can do, apart from watching for tell-tale signs. We can explain to our employers and governments that a surgeon's work is difficult, and different. They have to start realizing this, and stop taking advantage.

Airline-pilots and truck-drivers have their hours monitored, to make sure they've been rested. Presumably, insurance-companies would refuse payment, if they could prove otherwise. So why aren't surgeons being monitored and being prevented from over-working? It only needs some simple rules. Why are we liable to prosecution when it's already too late and then by unscrupulous 'ambulance-chasers'?

As for alcohol and drugs, it's not just airline pilots, train drivers, or chemical workers who are tested. In the science-fiction film Gattaca, a space agency's employees are automatically tested whenever they enter. A turnstile takes a tiny blood sample and checks their identity and health.

[14] It should be possible—it's anyway theoretically conceivable—to detect our own exhaustion through hormonal balance and biomarkers.

We surgeons need to fix this problem ourselves, before government steps in. We need to accept that there is a problem and that we are capable of fixing it ourselves, which already puts us two steps ahead of governments.

In the meantime, how can you remain "fit-for-task"?

Limit your administration, by employing a scribent [15]. Discipline your working hours, so you get a free day after a "night-on-call," and only a maximum of two nights-on-call per week [16, 17]. Devote some of your valuable time to sports. Up to 2.5 h of jogging a week at a slow or average pace would increase your life expectancy by 6.2 years for men and 5.6 years for women [18]. Make time to really listen to your patients. Learn what matters to them, as well as what's the matter with them. If you are good for your patients, they will be good for you. Lastly, keep the flame!! If there's light and humor and pleasure in what you do, then you're safe enough. But if you are dragging yourself along in the gloom, then you're already in trouble. Your balance is drifting into the red.

References

1. Van Dijk CN. Are we surgeons finding it all too much? Dealing with the pressures of our profession. JISAKOS. 2018;3(3):125–7.
2. McAulliffe W, Rohman M, Breer P, et al. Alcohol use and abuse in random samples of physicians. Am J Public Health. 1991;81:177–82.
3. Oreskovich MR, Kaups KL, Balch CM, et al. Prevalence of alcohol use disorders among American surgeons. Arch Surg. 2012;147:168–74.
4. Dimou FM, Eckelbarger D, Riall TS, et al. Surgeon burnout: a systematic review. J Am Coll Surg. 2016;222:1230–9.
5. Rollman BL, Mead LA, Wang NY, et al. Medical specialty and the incidence of divorce. N Engl J Med. 1997;336:800–3.
6. Dyrbye LN, Shanafelt TD, Balch CM, et al. Relationship between work-home conflicts and burnout among American surgeons. Arch Surg. 2011;146:211–7.
7. McHenry CR. In search of balance: a successful career, health, and family. Am J Surg. 2007;193:293–7.
8. Balch CM, Shanafelt TD, Sloan JA, et al. Distress and career satisfaction among 14 surgical specialties, comparing academic and private practice settings. Ann Surg. 2011a;254(1):558–68.
9. Zhang Y, Feng X. The relationship between job satisfaction, burnout, and turnover intention among physicians from urban state-owned medical institutions in Hubei, China: a cross-sectional study. BMC Health Serv Res. 2011;11:235.
10. Balch CM, Oreskovich MR, Dyrbye LN, et al. Personal consequences of malpractice lawsuits on American surgeons. J Am Coll Surg. 2011b;213(2):657–67.
11. Elton C. The Telegraph UK March 11, 2018. https://www.telegraph.co.uk/health-fitness/mind/depression-burn-trauma-exhaustion-inside-minds-doctors/.
12. Moran LJ. The anatomy of courage. London: Hachette UK; 1945.
13. Schnohr P, O'Keefe JH, Marott JL, et al. Dose of jogging and long-term mortality: the Copenhagen City Heart Study. J Am Coll Cardiol. 2015;65:411–9.
14. Gattaca, the movie. Direction Andrew Niccol. 1997. https://www.youtube.com/watch?v=q-loBxmnbl0.
15. Shultz CG, Holmstrom HL. The use of medical scribes in health care settings: a systematic review and future directions. J Am Board Fam Med. 2015;28(3):371–81. https://doi.org/10.3122/jabfm.2015.03.140224.
16. Shanafelt TD, Balch CM, Bechamps GJ, Russell T, Dyrbye L, Satele D, Collicott P, Novotny PJ, Sloan J, Freischlag JA. Burnout and career satisfaction among American surgeons. Ann Surg. 2009;250(3):463–71. https://doi.org/10.1097/SLA.0b013e3181ac4dfd.
17. Nicol AM, Botterill JS. On-call work and health: a review. Environ Health. 2004;3:15. https://doi.org/10.1186/1476-069X-3-15.
18. Schnohr P, Marott JL, Lange P, Jensen GB. Longevity in male and female joggers: the Copenhagen City heart study. Am J Epidemiol. 2013;177(7):683–9. https://doi.org/10.1093/aje/kws301.

Pseudoscience and False Avenues

9

Fares S. Haddad

As the world gets smaller, communication gets easier, the internet and social media dominate our world, and the pressure on physicians and the athletes that they are treating will continue to increase. The biggest risk moving forward is that rumour, marketing, conflicts and vested interests will stay a step ahead of the science that is really needed to help our athletes and to ensure their wellbeing.

The focus on performance and on success gets ever more fervent. Our athletes are bigger, stronger and faster than before. The pressure on them to train and to perform starts at a younger age. The rewards are greater. The energy of their sports and the collisions that ensue are getting to a point where they may be beyond the normal tolerance of human tissues.

We may be getting to a stage where we are able to, legally, or sometimes illegally, get athletes to gain the strength, speed and agility to destroy their skeletons at a young age. At the same time, the pressure to enhance performance, within the laws, or at the periphery of the laws and of ethical practice, and the pressure to deal with injuries expeditiously will continue to be so high that we are likely to be forced to seek and introduce new unproven interventions and treat our athletes in non-evidence-based ways.

In some cases, this will allow for quick recoveries and introduce new techniques and help the world sports community, but in others, it will damage a young vulnerable group of patients who are so driven that the dangers of experimental treatments are sometimes not considered.

The biggest danger of the next decade or two is that we will embrace pseudoscience where the need to do something, the need to do something new, and, indeed, the need to do something different from that being offered by others, will lead us down false avenues. We have seen that already, to a certain extent, with the use of biologics. Couching this in pseudoscience has led to stem cell interventions

F. S. Haddad (✉)
Division of Surgery, University College London, London, UK
e-mail: fsh@fareshaddad.net

© ISAKOS 2020   23
B. M. Devitt et al. (eds.), *The Future of Orthopaedic Sports Medicine*,
https://doi.org/10.1007/978-3-030-28976-8_9

worldwide where the evidence is limited, and, at other times, poor. Entire careers have been built around the use of various forms of PRP or other injectables. There are also questionable non-operative and operative protocols and interventions. There are very strong immovable expert views at all ends of the spectrum.

We often hide behind the fact that it is difficult to randomise and undertake high-level studies in our athletes and that may be indeed the case in some instances where standardisation is tough. On the other hand, unless we truly take a step back, collect robust data, subject ourselves and our athletes to genuine scientific scrutiny, and put safety above financial interests, it is likely that we will continue to do our athletes a disservice.

The danger is that the guru-led pseudoscientific application of apparently modern interventions that are attractive to referrers and attractive to athletes will continue to increase at a time when the edge required for high-level performance is so fine.

Orthopaedic sports medicine is at a very interesting time. Our speciality has grown at an exponential rate. We are faced with increasing numbers of athletes worldwide who have more information. We are faced with more data on training and performance. We should be very careful to analyse carefully and critically to truly build a genuine scientific evidence base that is free of conflicts. We should question the gurus, as practices are built on personality and often on pseudoscience. We should look after the next generation of athletes who are even more vulnerable than those who came before them. Whilst there will always inevitably be a role for expert-led interventions and for a compelling case series from someone who has an interest in a specific technique, and nowadays for consensus, which is sometimes an opportunity and sometimes a dangerous way of looking at the literature, we must try and raise the bar in terms of how we evaluate the interventions we apply to our athletes.

In brief, the dangers are that we are going to put our athletes under more and more pressure such that their skeletons cannot cope with the forces that are exerted through them. We will compound that further by being pressurised to allow them to perform too much at a young age while their skeletons are immature, and hence cause further damage, and also by applying interventions when they are fragile or injured that compromise them either in the short term or in the longer term, or both.

Orthopaedic sports medicine is yet to transition from an art to a science. There is a pretence that we must not be deluded by, and the introduction and the application of the true scientific method over the next two decades are critical. Alternatively, we may live in a happy fantasy world that fails those whom we are there to serve.

We'd Better Quit Now

James H. Lubowitz

Should we worry about the future of orthopedic sports medicine? Yes, we should.

First, I must disclose that I find the question sincerely appealing because I am prone to worry and habitually addicted to catastrophic thinking. (Much thanks–not–to the editors for playing to my these neuroses.) This may sound unfortunate but, actually, worst-case scenario thinking is a highly adaptive trait; if we can anticipate disaster, we can mitigate against loss and facilitate success. To that point, I need to type faster in case there is an earthquake.

So the question, "Should we worry about the future of orthopedic sports medicine?" is worthy. Yet having disclosed my tendency toward apprehension, I am actually bullish about the future of our field. Really, there is absolutely nothing to worry about. Everything will be fine. Wait, who are we kidding? There is everything to fear, we should absolutely fret, and it requires no stretch of the imagination to conjure our apocalyptic demise. But first, we have to avoid cataclysm.

Hear ye, hear ye orthopedic sports medicine specialists: disaster is imminent. Everywhere we turn, our opportunity for service, success, and fulfillment is obstructed, and our path is fraught with obstacles. Professional jealousy toward our humble ranks is rampant among our nonorthopedic "colleagues" (to use the term "loosely") and tendentiously simmers among even our orthopedic but non-sports medicine-specialized "frenemys." Burnout is high among our ranks, as we devote 100% of our energy to our patients plus 100% to our scholarship, and all the while, the bureaucrats and administrators demand and extract no less than another 100% (each) by creating inefficiency and mounting hurdles in the guise of "systems-based" practice. All right-minded practitioners recognize that the system is flawed. There is even a rumor among the rare pessimists and agnostics that there is no system at all. Competition among surgeons and scientists, as among institutions and societies, threatens cooperation among our best and our brightest. Ego and ambition

J. H. Lubowitz (✉)
Taos, NM, USA
e-mail: jlubowitz@kitcarson.net;
http://www.newmexicokneesurgery.com

© ISAKOS 2020 25
B. M. Devitt et al. (eds.), *The Future of Orthopaedic Sports Medicine*,
https://doi.org/10.1007/978-3-030-28976-8_10

result in temperamental behavior on the part of our educators, even after recess and a time-out, which sadly muddles their solipsistic messages, as does their poorly veiled demand to, "Look at me." Technology addles our brains and puts us at the mercy of billionaire youth who can write code (wearing hoodies no less), while information overload tempts us to crawl under the covers. Biologics is a Modern Prometheus not easily conquered (yet ever entertaining), and artificially intelligent robots will soon replace us and will replace our patients as well.

The future of orthopedic sports medicine is obviously bleak. There are signs everywhere. Our annual incomes have been generally reduced to a meager six figures, and while at least this gives us something to complain about, it is hard to find someone to listen (absent shackles and a strong sedative). Our ranks are growing more diverse, and if this remains unchecked, we could someday face outright heterogeneity. Our outcomes approach 100% good and excellent, yet we are distraught, confused, and frustrated because try as we might (and regardless of what we were told growing up), we just can't seem to be completely perfect. Our procedures grow less and less invasive, and our complication rates creep lower, but this is to the obvious detriment of our suture and bandage manufacturers, wound-care specialists, and the analgesics industry. Our research advances are beyond our wildest imagination, which just goes to show we are neither visionary nor creative.

Worst of all, orthopedic sports medicine specialists seem to always improve, but as we get better and better and smarter and smarter, we risk having our patients get so healthy and heal and perform so well that we might successfully put ourselves right out of existence. To be clear, our faithful endeavors to prevent illness and injury, improve safety, and promote the public health will result in the ultimate demise of our field.

The future of orthopedic sports medicine is bleak. We are popular, affluent, successful, savvy, energetic, sophisticated, advanced, empathetic, minimally invasive, altruistic, scholarly, distinct, ever improving, and of service to mankind. If we don't quit now, it is inevitable that we could continue the risk of making our world a better place.

We'd better quit now.

Academic Integrity and the God of Data

11

Nathan White

"In God we trust, all others must bring data." Commonly attributed to the statistician William Deming [1], this remark implores us to prove our work beyond relying on trust, opinion, and personal assurance. The way to do so, it would seem, is with data. But what if the data we rely on is wrong, misleading, or misinterpreted[1]?

I woke recently to news that Harvard University had retracted 31 papers on a topic indirectly related to Orthopaedic Sports Medicine [2]. After more than a decade of attempts, a prominent researcher's work was unable to be replicated and had been denounced as fraud. It brought to mind another example, that of Andrew Wakefield [3], which risked immense damage to the most vulnerable in our society and abused the trust placed in the medical profession.

Fortunately, few of our colleagues are so dishonest. Yet data is famously open to interpretation. In a study published in *Nature* [4], 29 teams of researchers analysed the same data set, seeking to determine whether football (soccer) players with dark skin received more red cards than those with light skin. Even with a seemingly straightforward exercise, there was considerable difference in how teams interpreted exactly the same information. Even among teams agreeing on the overall result, there was large variation in both the methods they chose and, ultimately, the results they found.

Once published, bad research is difficult and time consuming to make right. Fiction disperses throughout the profession and into the wider community, undifferentiated from fact. It may be studied and built upon by academics acting in good faith. Now, more than ever, there is the temptation to promote new techniques, and

---

[1] The earliest print reference to this saying, referring to it as a 'well-recognised cliché', comes not from Deming but from a 1978 Congressional hearing into passive smoking, where it was used to argue against proposals to limit smoking in public places, as evidence of harm was lacking.

N. White (✉)
Park Clinic Orthopaedics, Melbourne, VIC, Australia

© ISAKOS 2020
B. M. Devitt et al. (eds.), *The Future of Orthopaedic Sports Medicine*,
https://doi.org/10.1007/978-3-030-28976-8_11

the technology to reach an enormous audience. Pages are filled, treatments commenced, and those involved may be headed towards disappointment.

Clearly, there is a need for transparent, high-quality data to justify what we do. However, data by itself is not God. Or, perhaps, it's a god styled after Greek mythology; powerful but fickle, imperfect and fallible, and it won't always be there to guide us. We are wise to approach it with a clear mind and show leadership in how it is interpreted and applied. There is equally a duty to ensure that helpful research is disseminated to clinicians and patients in an accessible and timely manner but without embellishment or hyperbole. Researchers should not seek to become spin doctors, but our views must be heard for our ideas to flourish. How can we do this effectively, ethically, in an era when complex ideas are reduced to 140 characters or less, and whoever shouts the loudest wins?

Somewhat paradoxically, given the opening statement in this chapter, I believe the solution to these worries lies largely in trust. Data is essential, but it is only one pillar of research. A new treatment, proven beyond doubt, will never realise its potential unless it is trusted. Clinicians are cautious of agenda-driven evidence, serving to prop up ideas rather than to illuminate. Likewise, patients are not naïve to the fact that there is potential for controversy and bias in medical research. Our behaviour as a scientific community must be above reproach. We must act with integrity and cultivate trust.

There is an understanding that contradictory evidence will occasionally emerge, that treatments can change over time, and that hopefully results will improve. When we conduct ourselves well, there is forgiveness on offer. Balancing the limitations of our hard-won data, there remains a good deal of trust in our profession. This should be safeguarded above all else because while data can provide proof beyond trust, it is imperfect. And without trust, we would simply be talking to, and for, ourselves.

References

1. United States. Congress. House. Committee on Agriculture. Subcommittee on Tobacco. Effect of smoking on nonsmokers: hearing before the subcommittee on tobacco. United States congress house committee on agriculture. Subcommittee on tobacco. Washington: U.S. Government Printing Office; 1978. p. 345.
2. Kolata G. Harvard calls for retraction of dozens of studies by noted cardiac researcher. New York: New York Times; 2018. https://www.nytimes.com/2018/10/15/health/piero-anversa-fraud-retractions.html
3. Retraction: ileal lymphoid nodular hyperplasia, non-specific colitis, and pervasive developmental disorder in children. Lancet. 2010;375:445.
4. Silberzahn R, Uhlmann EL. Crowdsourced reseach: many hands make tight work. Nature. 2015;526(7572):189–91. https://doi.org/10.1038/526189a.

Research Funding: Finding a Balance

Fernando Gómez Verdejo

In the practice of Orthopedic sports medicine, there is an eagerness to conduct research underpinned by a desire to make improvements in our practice and ultimately generate an impact on the treatment and recovery of our patients. Desire is not enough—research requires funding for both the hours people invest as well as premises and equipment.

The ongoing challenge is that there is a lack of understanding regarding the importance of research by some of the parties potentially funding it—perhaps because the results and benefits of research are rarely immediate and even more rarely profitable. This is especially true in developing, or "newly industrialized" countries, where research stimulus is of exceptional importance.

Funding can be roughly categorized into private and public, and there seems to be a growing gap between the former and the latter in respect to enthusiasm when it comes to financing research projects. The trend in many developing countries is of public budget cuts. This gap is not left unfilled—industry-based funding organizations frequently will step in to replace it. In privately funded research, commercial gain can threaten to trump the benefits for patients.

The patterns and trends in private-based research give some indication of this. There have been multiple recent studies in the field of orthopedics and other related specialties linking commercial party funding to studies that as a whole tend to present positive conclusions more often than their public or non-profit-funded counterparts. Likewise, private-funding contracts have been previously reported to prevent or at the very least delay the publication of studies whose results were deemed to not be in the best interest of the financing party, not to mention cases in which ongoing research projects have been completely halted, as preliminary results were unfavorable to the sponsor. Moreover, it has been found and documented that there is a statistically significant difference in pro-industry results when comparing studies with public financing versus those that were endorsed by a private company.

F. G. Verdejo (✉)
Instituto Nacional de Rehabilitación, Mexico City, Mexico

© ISAKOS 2020
B. M. Devitt et al. (eds.), *The Future of Orthopaedic Sports Medicine*,
https://doi.org/10.1007/978-3-030-28976-8_12

While these facts do not constitute evidence for bias in every single case, they do present a reality that if extrapolated to a setting as the one described previously, where public and non-profit funding become virtually nonexistent, it sets the tone for a reality in which our practice could end up mainly benefiting a commercial organization or a group of organizations rather than our patients.

Industry-based research may, in some instances, completely outweigh publicly funded research, simply because it is more attractive for governmental institutions to divert funding to programs that render more immediate results. This is particularly attractive for developing countries, but it could have dire consequences for patients in these regions due to the biases that can, at times, come with privately funded research.

While we should regard this concern as one of the utmost importance, it would be unwise to entertain the thought of private funding in itself as being a crutch for development of new techniques and technologies. It should be rather regarded as an element in a balanced equation, one that includes government institutions and non-profit organizations operating in newly industrialized regions.

Finally, as we look forward to taking actions to solve this matter, there is much that can be learnt from initiatives and programs in more developed countries. For example, the implementation of publicly funded national and regional joint registries, a trend that has mainly impacted the field of arthroplasty, but that is also present in the field of orthopedic sports medicine, as exemplified by the Norwegian Cruciate Ligament Registry and the Swedish Anterior Cruciate Ligament Registry. These systems that currently exist in a handful of countries greatly promote data collection and publicly funded research that unequivocally support an evidence-based practice.

These types of initiatives are practically unheard-of in most developing regions. A positive first step would be to introduce these systems to provide an alternative option to the current model of simply publicly versus privately funded research.

From Science to Daily Practice: A Huge Gap! The Example of Meniscus Surgery

13

Philippe Beaufils

It is well accepted that our practice should be based on evidence-based medicine (EBM). EBM is promoted as conscientious, explicit and judicious use of current best evidence in the decision making about individualised patients care. However, it is often viewed as the Holy Grail. But when meniscus surgery is considered, there is a huge gap between scientific evidence and daily practice. In recent times, there has been a vogue to 'save the meniscus', which has promoted repair or preservation in the meniscus whatever the type of the meniscus lesion, traumatic or degenerative.

Degenerative meniscal tears have garnered much attention in the literature, with nine randomised controlled trials (RCTs) having been performed since 2003. All of these studies except one [1] concluded that the outcomes of non-operative treatment are similar to those of primary arthroscopic meniscectomy. The risk of cross-over from non-operative treatment to arthroscopic meniscectomy at 1-year follow-up ranges from 0% to 30%. The obvious consequence is that non-operative treatment should be proposed as a first-line treatment, expecting a significant decrease in the meniscectomy rate. However, and as examples, at the same time, meniscectomy rate dramatically increased in Denmark, especially in older patients [2], and slightly decreased in France but only in younger patients.

In traumatic meniscal tears, there are stronger criteria to support meniscal repair. Indeed, there are certain types of tear that are amenable to repair and have promising results—vertical and longitudinal tears, tears located in the vascular zone and acute tears; these tear configurations typically represent 25% of meniscal lesions encountered. However, the meniscus repair rate, even if it is getting slightly better, remains far lower than 25%, especially when associated with ACL reconstruction.

P. Beaufils (✉)
Department of Orthopaedics and Traumatology, Centre Hospitalier de Versailles (CHV), Versailles, France
e-mail: pbeaufils@ch-versailles.fr

© ISAKOS 2020

B. M. Devitt et al. (eds.), *The Future of Orthopaedic Sports Medicine*, https://doi.org/10.1007/978-3-030-28976-8_13

It clearly appears that EBM alone is not able to deeply and rapidly influence our daily practice. Thus, is it really relevant to a sports medicine speciality where outcome assessment is generally very subtle and patient dependent?

Several factors could explain the gap:

1. The Scientific Value of RCTs: RCTs, despite being some of the highest level of evidence, do contain some weaknesses. The selection bias is probably the most relevant. Does a very selected sample of patients (which is often the consequence of a strict protocol of randomization) reflect the global population? This is easily pointed out by readers who do not agree with conclusions and prefer to underline the weaknesses rather than the strengths of a study (contamination bias).
2. The Myth: 'I've always done it this wasy and it works. Why should I change?'
3. The Surgery First: As stated by Bruce Reider in the 2016 AJSM editorial 'To cut or not to cut…', We, as surgeons, are formatted to think surgery first and when surgical or non-operative management are in balance, our spontaneous tendency is to go for surgery.
4. The Technique: Some techniques require a learning curve or are supposed to be more difficult or more time consuming than well-known and accepted techniques. Is it obvious that a lateral meniscus repair is more demanding than a lateral meniscectomy?
5. The Society: Patients (who reflect our society) are active partners in the decision-making process. The overuse of imaging tools may lead to excessive surgical procedures. The demand for rapid answers or recovery may lead to a questionable decision. Recovery after meniscectomy in traumatic tears is said to be faster than after repair. Is it really true? Non-operative treatment in degenerative meniscus lesions is often seen as a non-treatment, while meniscectomy is an active answer, even if not necessary.
6. Economic Issues: Health care insurance systems really influence daily practice, depending on many factors. Whatever the country, they are unfortunately often based on old, well-established managements and do not take into account more modern ways, even if they are 'scientifically' proven.

How could the gap be reduced? Consensus is the probably the most appropriate way and is the reason why ESSKA published a Consensus on Degenerative Meniscus Lesion management in 2017 [3]. A Consensus is not a Systematic Review of the literature. The Consensus is a mix of EBM (including Systematic Review) and clinical expertise. The Consensus does not only include leaders and pioneers but also daily practitioners. Finally, the Consensus is an independent process involving all the specialities of the same field, which may facilitate a rapid appropriation in our daily practice. To conclude, we can claim that EBM is of course necessary but not sufficient to convince the orthopaedic and sports medicine community to adopt new ways!

References

1. Gauffin H, Tagesson S, Meunier A, Magnusson H, Kvist J. Knee arthroscopic surgery is beneficial to middle-aged patients with meniscal symptoms: a prospective, randomised, single-blinded study. Osteoarthr Cartil. 2014;22(11):1808–16.
2. Thorlund JB, Hare KB, Lohmander LS. Large increase in arthroscopic meniscus surgery in the middle-aged and older population in Denmark from 2000 to 2011. Acta Orthop. 2014;85(3):287–92.
3. Beaufils P, Becker R, Kopf S, et al. Surgical management of degenerative meniscus lesions: the 2016 ESSKA meniscus consensus. Joints. 2017;5(2):59–69.

Living on the Edge

14

Asbjørn Årøen

Infectious diseases have always been a major health challenge, which can also give rise to major musculoskeletal problems. In medical school, older professors told us about problems related to tuberculosis infections in bone and how difficult these infections were to treat. In my 26 years of work, I have been involved in only one case of bone tuberculosis, although such cases remind us that infectious diseases remain in our midst.

Our modern society has succeeded in many ways in minimizing orthopedic infections through progress in sterilization practices and operating room procedures. Infections still occur, particularly in association with joint replacement and other replacement procedures as well as ligament surgery. The latest approach is to load a graft with local antibiotics or to liberally utilize such antibiotics during a procedure; however, there is extremely little evidence of the effectiveness of this approach, which may possibly promote the development of multi-resistant bacteria. The use of this approach indicates an ignorance of threats to general health among my colleagues, which is an issue that greatly concerns me, and I am uncertain that even well-conducted research that proves them wrong will turn the wheel toward safer practices with respect to the use of local antibiotics.

Sports medicine is one of the most profitable fields in the Western world; as a result, orthopedic surgery is an extremely popular choice for medical students in most countries with major private health care.

Our Earth is overcrowded, and the planet will surely retaliate; among the potential means of retaliation, an epidemic infectious disease might be one of the most effective ways of reducing the number of inhabitants on the Earth.

A. Årøen (✉)
Department of Orthopedic Surgery, Institute of Clinical Medicine, Akershus University Hospital, Campus Ahus University of Oslo, Oslo, Norway
e-mail: asbjorn.aroen@medisin.uio.no

© ISAKOS 2020
B. M. Devitt et al. (eds.), *The Future of Orthopaedic Sports Medicine*,
https://doi.org/10.1007/978-3-030-28976-8_14

Although we are living on the edge with respect to this particular topic, there is hope if we can maintain the balance between ourselves and the bacterial microenvironment. In this context, orthopedic surgery must also face the challenge of finding ways to prevent the evolution of infection other than merely increasing antibiotic loads administered in hospitals.

Currently, there are few new effective antibiotics in the pipeline, and multiresistant bacteria are most commonly found in countries where regulations governing the use of such antibiotics are relatively flexible.

The Last Generation of Doctors

Brett A. Fritsch

The future is an exciting place. What I worry about is what relevance we may have in it. The machines are coming.

Now, before you envision Skynet and malicious terminators, let's be clear—it won't be malicious machines that replace us, it will be competent ones. When I say machines, what I really mean are intelligent algorithms that are far more effective at diagnosing our patients, forming the treatment plans with the highest chance of success, and eventually becoming better at delivering these interventions than we are. We won't be eliminated, just redundant.

Medicine is essentially complex pattern recognition. We take a patients history, add some clinical findings, and combine it with the necessary investigations to make a diagnosis. We then combine our acquired medical knowledge with feedback we observe from the patients we have treated in order to refine our treatment plan for the next patients. It's a slow loop of gradually improving pattern recognition.

Computers love patterns, and they are very good at finding them. The limiting factors are computing power and the size of the data set they have to examine. Both are growing at exponential rates. A supercomputer of 20 years ago is now sitting in your pocket, and the rate of improvement is only accelerating. Recently, it was projected that a computer would surpass the processing power of the human brain sometime around 2023—it happened last week. The world's fastest supercomputer, the Summit, runs at 200 Petaflops, which is 200,000 trillion calculations per second. A calculation that takes 1 min for this machine takes your desktop PC 30 years, and in 10 years' time, that power will be sitting in your pocket (or more to the point, in your patients' pocket).

Data sets are growing at the same rate. Electronic medical records, national registries, and compulsory patient-reported outcomes are all becoming

B. A. Fritsch (✉)
Sydney, NSW, Australia
e-mail: brett@brettfritsch.com.au

© ISAKOS 2020
B. M. Devitt et al. (eds.), *The Future of Orthopaedic Sports Medicine*,
https://doi.org/10.1007/978-3-030-28976-8_15

standard. Apple watches, Fitbits, and the multitude of other wearables are tracking almost all aspects of our physiology, and our own records of our life via social media give a far better picture of how we are feeling than any formal PROM questionnaire (a recent study of Facebook data showed that if you have "liked" more than ten things, then the FB algorithm can predict your future likes better than your family. If it is more than 30, then FB knows you better than your spouse does!).

We are rapidly quantifying what it is to be human. Linking these data sets to the computational abilities of machines like Summit and its descendants will allow health-related pattern recognition far beyond that of a mere human being.

These algorithms will be self-learning, and in fact, they already are. In 2006, Deep Blue defeated Gary Kasparov in a series of chess matches by simply outcalculating him (at a mere 200 million calculations per second—less than your iPhone's capabilities). In 2016, Lee Sedol, the greatest exponent of the game of Go, was defeated by AlphaGo, an algorithm that used millions of historical games of Go to identify successful patterns of moves and to apply them to its next move in real time. Less than 18 months later AlphaGoZero defeated the same algorithm 100:0 using general reinforcement learning algorithms, a process of providing it with the rules of Go, the goals of go, and a process for learning its own successful strategies. Within 72 h, AlphaGoZero was the best Go playing "intelligence" on the Earth, with no further human intervention and no historical data required. Almost every week a similar new example of AI capability is reported, and medicine is ripe for its application.

This ability to learn, with the ever (exponentially) increasing computational power, and massive data sets will initially augment our profession, but it's hard to see how it will not replace it.

I know what you are thinking—"this will never happen"—well, it already is. Imaging algorithms are more accurate than radiologists at examining mammograms and chest X-rays for cancer, and skin cancers can be detected by similar systems with greater accuracy than by dermatologists. In 2017, an algorithm sat and passed the general Chinese medical licensing exam, scoring 96 points above the required pass mark.

What about your certainty that "patients will always want to see a real doctor." I'm not sure that's the case either. If your children are like mine, they are already quite comfortable taking friend suggestions from Facebook, and song suggestions from iTunes, and they seem to listen to Google Home and Alexa more than they listen to me sometimes. I don't think this generation will have any problem taking their medical advice, and eventually treatment, from a system other than the traditional doctor, particularly when it is faster, more accessible, cheaper, and ultimately more accurate, than the human alternative. The fears we have about the downside of new technologies all tend to disappear in the face of competence and convenience.

So my worry (or hope?) is that the future of sports medicine will not even need us. For a period, we may remain as manual technicians, delivering the surgeries that are predicted by the Artificial Intelligence (AI) to have the highest chance of success, but eventually, even this role will be replaced. In the last 20 years, we have gone from using paper maps to navigate our cars, to GPS to be guided, to the threshold of handing the steering wheel over to the algorithms altogether. This transition has occurred because, at every step, the technology results in increased accuracy, convenience, safety, and result in achieving the goal. I don't see why our pathway will be, or should be, any different.

The Future of Orthopaedic Sports Medicine: It's the Human Connection

16

Scott Schaffner

Rapid technological advances, automation, digital and cloud-based technologies are commonplace in everything from consumer goods to the operating room, and orthopedic sports medicine is seeing the benefit. New training and treatment methods such as virtual reality and bioinductive implants in surgery are enhancing not only the effectiveness of a surgeon's craft but also the pace at which patients are healing and getting back to their lives.

Moreover, we are currently witnessing a resurgence in collective health consciousness globally. With this, two trends are likely to emerge. First, the shift from addressing performance deficiencies (injuries) to instead a focus on performance optimization, returning patients to their pre-injury state. The second trend being surgeries and the tools for those surgeries that are more closely tailored to specific patient needs. Both trends point to one thing—reenergizing the human connection in orthopedic sports medicine.

Adopting a tailored, human-centered approach presents the challenge of being able to scale performance for the many needs of the patient, from both a clinical and financial perspective. As medical device manufacturers, we must carefully consider where to invest and where to focus our research so that the global majority benefits from the advances in orthopedic sports medicine.

Similarly, when looking at the technologies that allow for the shift to performance optimization, we again have to ensure access on a global scale. Resources, surgical technique and surgeon needs vary from one region to another, and we must understand regional and local differences in customer needs, as it gives the most accurate perspective of the future possibilities.

Investing in the right technologies and procedures alongside a solid portfolio is key to a configurable patient-specific solution. This works only if our collective focus

S. Schaffner (✉)
Smith+Nephew, Andover, MA, USA
e-mail: Scott.Schaffner@smith-nephew.com

© ISAKOS 2020   41
B. M. Devitt et al. (eds.), *The Future of Orthopaedic Sports Medicine*,
https://doi.org/10.1007/978-3-030-28976-8_16

remains on the patient as an end user and the medical professional who enables patients to return to pre-injury performance with the support of our solutions.

We depend on our close relationships with leading surgeons and medical professionals worldwide to help us understand the gaps and needs in the market. This knowledge and working closely with the medical community allows us to invest in the right technologies that will shape the future and help improve patients' lives. In the same way that we rely on the relationships with surgeons and providers to help us understand how we can stay at the forefront of innovation, our employees help us deliver on our promise and allow us to stay competitive. Tapping into the knowledge and experience of more than 16,000 global employees makes Smith+Nephew a better company.

Ensuring the relationship between technology and human work in harmony is paramount. Innovating for the sake of technology must be viewed critically. It is more than having the trendiest technology; it is having a purpose-driven solution that allows for performance optimization in a configurable surgical approach. Where technology is advancing, so too must the people; where one develops, so does the other and vice versa. So, while we talk about the future of sports medicine and the possibilities and risks, we should never lose sight of the people that make it all happen and the patients whose lives we are all working to improve.

17

The Meniscus Is the Most Important Piece of the Knee

Nicolas Pujol

"Take it out. Take it all out. Even it is not torn, take it out." These famous words allegedly spoken by Smillie over 40 years ago should stay in the mind of every orthopedic knee surgeon because of their ludicrous meanings and drastic consequences.

The meniscus is the most important piece of the knee. When it is gone, it is over.

Meniscectomy is still one of the most popular and frequent orthopedic procedures in the world. But long-term results, even with arthroscopic "partial" meniscectomy, are not so good, and the concept of meniscal preservation has, therefore, progressed over the years. However, the meniscectomy rate remains too high despite robust scientific publications that report the advantages of meniscal repair or nonremoval of the meniscus in traumatic tears and nonremoval rather than meniscectomy in degenerative meniscal lesions. It is worrying to note the considerable gap between these publications, this knowledge, and daily practice. It is even more concerning to note that this tendency is consistent over time and is adopted on all continents. There are still many contrived and plainly incorrect reasons for orthopedic surgeons to perform meniscectomies rather than carry out meniscal repairs. All of these need to be discussed, and they must be deleted of one's subconscious:

1. "I think that meniscectomy is a safe, quick, and easy procedure for me; so, it will be the same for the patient": Wrong! There are some publications comparing meniscectomy and meniscal repair, especially on the lateral side. Time to return to sports is higher after lateral meniscectomy, and sometimes, the patient never returns to his/her preinjury level of participation.
2. "Meniscal repair procedure has a long learning curve and is only dedicated to few simple lesions located in the vascular area of the meniscus. The rate of failure is high": Wrong! All the literature reviews of meniscal repair bring together

N. Pujol (✉)
Department of Orthopedic Surgery, Centre Hospitalier de Versailles, Le Chesnay, France
e-mail: npujol@ch-versailles.fr

© ISAKOS 2020   43
B. M. Devitt et al. (eds.), *The Future of Orthopaedic Sports Medicine*,
https://doi.org/10.1007/978-3-030-28976-8_17

recent papers with modern techniques and old papers with devices and techniques that are not in use anymore. So, the overall rate of failure and subsequent meniscectomy is around 20%. When looking to the recent literature using modern devices, techniques, and selected indications, this rate is rather close to 7–10%. There are many repairable meniscal lesions, not only the classic vertical longitudinal lesion. Root lesions, radial lesions, and horizontal cleavages are often repairable.

3. Patient and society: "I saw professional athletes on the television and they returned to preinjury level quickly after a meniscectomy, so please Doctor: do the same for me, even if I am not a professional athlete and even if my lesion is repairable": Wrong! There are specific indications of surgery in the professional athlete that should not be extended to the global population.

Furthermore, there are some meniscal lesions that can be left in situ without any surgical treatment. No surgery can be recommended in many cases. Degenerative meniscal lesions are common in the middle-aged patients, often associated with early osteoarthritis. In such cases, the first treatment is the treatment of OA and not the treatment of the degenerative meniscal lesions, even if it is root lesions. During ACL reconstruction, many partial or small complete lesions of the posterior part of the lateral meniscus can be left alone without meniscectomy or repair. We should not overtreat our patients.

It is definitely time to change the paradigm in the management of the meniscus. Meniscectomy should never be the first-line choice. Meniscal lesions are not all repairable, of course. But all repairable meniscal lesions must be repaired. A lot of meniscal lesions need to be operated on, sometimes by doing a meniscectomy. But some of them do not require any surgery.

My Wishes for the Next Decade Are:

The establishment of a world consensus for the treatment of meniscal lesions, respected and used by every surgeon.

All patients treated with the best indication, depending on the type of lesion often meniscal preservation, often repair, sometimes without surgery, and at the end (as rare as possible): a partial meniscectomy.

Is Medicine Now a Science or Still an Art?

18

Philippe Landreau

During my residency in Paris, I spent some time with my mentor, Professor Jacques Witvoët. At this time, he was one of the pre-eminent figures in this field, and his reputation attracted many young surgeons from France and abroad. His experience and rigor were well known, and his practical education was established on three pillars:

The first one was the *practical teaching on clinical cases*. All patients' cases were discussed during a weekly meeting, which gathered all physicians in the surgical department. The patient was present at the beginning of the meeting, when a history of the presenting complaint and past medical history were taken and a clinical examination performed. The patient was asked to explain his/her expectations of treatment and was then asked to leave the room. The case was then discussed, argued and validated by the surgical team under the guidance of our mentor. Finally, the patient was asked to return to the room, and the case was explained along with the therapeutic plan. In addition to this crucial meeting, each patient who was operated on was once again discussed with the "boss" at a postoperative meeting the day after surgery, a debriefing session, if you will. I think I never learned so much in my life than during these sessions about individualized patient evaluation and treatment; "*à la carte*" care at its finest.

The second pillar was based on a sound knowledge of the literature. A journal club was established where each resident and assistant were expected to present a recent paper related to our clinical practice. Our mentor didn't speak much English, and this is probably the reason why he didn't disseminate his experience internationally. Nonetheless, he was aware of his limited coverage and knew that the new generation needed to have access and to be exposed to a wide variety of literature, especially the international, English-speaking experts.

P. Landreau (✉)
DXBone, Bone and Joint Excellence Center, Dubai, UAE

B. M. Devitt et al. (eds.), *The Future of Orthopaedic Sports Medicine*,
https://doi.org/10.1007/978-3-030-28976-8_18

The third pillar was the value of experience. His own experience, which was tremendous, was shared with us as young surgeons. Nevertheless, he expounded on the importance of gaining your own experience and getting exposure to complex cases. He emphasized that books and articles are certainly important but less so than the experience we gain from our routine practice.

When I reflect on my formative years in orthopedics from my current perspective, I realize that my mentor, even in those early days, was teaching us evidence-based medicine (EBM), even before that term was coined. He was ahead of his time. In essence, EBM is the assembly and integration of clinical experience, coupled with the patient outcomes, which is supported by the best available research. The collection of these elements should lead to the best practice for patient care. There is no doubt that EBM is a real advancement for our daily practice. On a positive note, it allows us not to be unduly influenced by expert opinion alone, as it was in the past. But unfortunately, there has been a recent tendency to stick too rigidly to literature-based evidence at the expense of personal experience. Understandably, a young, inexperienced practitioner, working alone, unaided by senior colleagues will lean on the literature, which is so readily available nowadays. Nevertheless, as surgeons, we must build our own experience based on our own patients' outcome and not simply what the literature tells us.

An excessive reliance on the literature is dangerous. Firstly, it is not always synonymous with the truth. Consider a recent study on systematic reviews and meta-analyses which revealed that less than one-third of the studies included level 1 and 2 evidence [1]. Secondly, each patient is unique, which is not always relevant to the cohort described in level 1 studies. Furthermore, algorithms for decision making are only guidelines, which can be useful at a basic level for the care of a single patient. Therefore, my worry is that in the future of the orthopedics and sports medicine, we will follow EBM blindly and forget to look at the patient sitting directly in front of us.

Listen to your patients, use your own experience (or the experience of your mentor), and support your decision with the available recent literature. It is a subtle distinction but explains why medicine is not simply a science but is still considered an art.

Reference

1. DiSilvestro KJ, Tjoumakaris FP, Maltenfort MG, Spindler KP, Freedman KB. Systematic reviews in sports medicine. Am J Sports Med. 2016;44(2):533–8.

Let's Get Back to Basics

Jérôme Murgier

19.1 No Scrum... No Win

Like on a rugby field, respecting the basics is fundamental to success. The famous quote "no scrum, no win" could easily be applied to the sports medicine field... and probably to life.

The philosophy of "sticking to basics" refers to retaining and adhering to fundamental skills, knowledge and teaching—sticking to governing principles while we embrace the benefit of new technologies. This approach will prevent the disappearance of our specialty, which is progressively being challenged.

Whatever technology brings to us, the fact remains an ACL tear will be the same in 200 years as it is now, and the Lachman test will be required to confirm the diagnosis. The trend, increasingly so, is to do less physical examinations and rely more heavily on modern X-rays or MRIs to make the diagnosis; but as sports surgeons "sticking to basics" means continuing to perform the complete physical examination to enable the detection of specific instability (e.g. hyperlaxity, high grade pivot shift) requiring a specific procedure. "Sticking to basics" also means that we should not forget the "orthopaedic language", whether it is biomechanical, anatomical or ortho-biological. These original concepts remain valid and will continue so in the future. For instance, in 1879, the French surgeon Paul Segond discovered the anterolateral ligament, only for it to be rediscovered 150 years later. This represents a missed opportunity to learn from our predecessors. The temptation to rely heavily on modern tests and recent publications is high. However, basic principles will remain pivotal to critical decision-making processes. Imparting these principles to junior doctors is our duty to ensure the protection of our profession from the vulnerabilities that all of modern medicine faces. Educating our trainees helps preserve our sense of togetherness and strengthens the orthopaedic community by forming collegial alliances.

J. Murgier (✉)
Toulouse, France

© ISAKOS 2020
B. M. Devitt et al. (eds.), *The Future of Orthopaedic Sports Medicine*,
https://doi.org/10.1007/978-3-030-28976-8_19

Moreover, the patient-doctor relationship has evolved over time with patients self-diagnosing through online forums; however, patients continue to seek empathy, understanding and kindness. The Hippocratic Oath is a great example of "sticking to basics", this oath provides a higher degree of humanism in dealing with the needs, well-being and interests of people when compared to other codes of conduct and we should not stop using it; it is part of our history and our culture.

Like facing your opponent on the rugby field, the orthopaedic sports society faces its own risks and threats. The future of our profession is vulnerable to the influx of new technologies and to the influence of other specialties (physiotherapy, osteopathy, etc.). Consequently, some patients are no longer immediately referred to orthopaedic surgeons even after an ACL tear (i.e. recent publications highlight the success of rehabilitation program in ACL tears without reconstruction). The role of the surgeon is challenged and will continue to be challenged by the advent of technological, biological and commercial innovations.

The sports medicine specialty benefits from the use of modern technologies to obtain the best results for patients. Be it the use of robotics or artificial intelligence, these innovations will modify the surgeon's role and alter our activity. It is foreseeable that in the future, a robot will be able to do an ACL reconstruction with perfectly positioned tunnels at a rapid rate and with good outcomes. What will the role of the surgeon be here? Will the surgeon become a technician? Or will the technician replace the surgeon? It is possible that the surgeon will take on a more passive role to oversee the operation and intervene only if something goes wrong. Moreover, it is likely that new technology may allow patients to avoid surgery altogether. This change could potentially reinvent the environment we work in and hopefully improve patient outcomes. Surgeons will need to adapt to facilitate alternate methods, otherwise face the prospect of falling behind and losing the scrum.

The biological revolution has already begun. One of the best examples is the multi-faceted use of PRP in sports medicine, which is quickly becoming a popular alternative for treating tendonitis, muscle injuries, cartilage defects or even ligamentous pain. Sport physicians often mediate the process with the involvement of radiologists who inject the treatment. Orthopaedic surgeons are therefore excluded from this treatment pathway. If we look at the future and think about similar cases of biological advances, we can anticipate that "targeted" stem cells might be available to act specifically in the damaged area to treat intra-articular tears without surgery. An ACL tear could potentially be treated by an injection of ACL-specific stem cells directly into the joint. In this scenario, the orthopaedic surgeon would not even be required to see these patients. More than ever, surgeons need to be the agents of change or risk getting benched.

Large pharmaceutical companies have already begun to finance new innovations with mounting pressure on medical practitioners to use these new "miraculous" products. The price of innovation is anticipated to continue to rise. Furthermore, this will strengthen the already popular argument to "avoid surgery", as seen in the treatment of inflammatory arthropathies. Innovations offering non-surgical interventions may be more enticing to patients, especially since they are readily available from professionals willing to offer them. This combined with funding from companies that profit from the success of these methods will threaten the role of surgeons. It is easy to imagine an advertisement for the treatment of ACL injuries without surgery by injecting "ACL-specific stem cells". If this proves to be scientifically sound and beneficial, then we need to be the agents of change.

Importantly, new innovations still require scientific evidence to justify their use as a superior alternative to surgery. We must continue to position ourselves as scientific authorities to address the foreseeable challenges ahead. Moreover, as we have seen with PRP or double-bundle ACL reconstructions, new ideas are not necessarily the best ones. While we should embrace new technologies with excitement and a healthy dose of critical appraisal, we should never forget the strength of basics principles. "No scrum, no win"… Let's get back to basics!

We Should Be Worried, About Being Worried!

Matthew Brick

It is my observation that in the operating room, we should be worried about being worried. What are the synonyms for worry? To be concerned, be anxious, agonize, brood, dwell on, panic, lose sleep, become worked up and get flustered over a problem either real or imagined. The underlying emotion here is fear. Fear comes in many forms in the operating room, and we have all been there: audible arterial injury, an ACL tunnel blowing out, losing fixation at a critical moment and equipment unavailability at a crucial time.

How do we react? Informing the team 'I am anxious' or 'I am afraid' is often not in our immediate repertoire of responses. It is far more common for fear to come out sideways as anger. Anger seems more comfortable and authoritative. Everyone in the room knows it, from the scrub team to the anaesthetist, the circulating nurse, the resident and fellow. But what are the benefits of this approach? I would argue there are none.

What happens to the surgeon? The breadth of our awareness is lost. We drill down in our focus to what we believe to be most important in that moment and can rapidly lose the bigger picture. We lose the subtle feel of our fingertips. The arthroscopic instruments are the extension of our tactile sensation, crucial to fluid, atraumatic surgery. We start to get rough: sutures snap and anchors bend, and articular cartilage is knocked and damaged. We simply are no longer giving the patient our best.

What happens to our team? They are fearful too: fearful of us. The astute observations of experienced staff are no longer conveyed. Our team also loses their own awareness, and if errors are seen, in self-preservation mode, they are more likely to keep it to themselves. Valuable skills in the room are lost, as team members become more concerned about keeping their heads down and avoiding being the focus of our temper rather than maximising the result for the patient asleep on the table.

M. Brick (✉)
Orthosports, North Shore, Auckland, New Zealand
e-mail: mat@orthosports.co.nz

© ISAKOS 2020   51
B. M. Devitt et al. (eds.), *The Future of Orthopaedic Sports Medicine*,
https://doi.org/10.1007/978-3-030-28976-8_20

We each have our own telltale signs that things are not going to plan. I soak through my scrub top with sweat, needing a change after the case. I go quiet and my conversation stops. However, a 30-year meditation habit has saved me from the angry outburst. First thing in the morning, 20 minutes spent sitting quietly and focussing on my breathing serves as a fresh start. Observing one's own thoughts and feelings gradually becomes an easy habit and being able to empty our mind of scrambled, anxious thoughts very useful in a tense situation.

My trips to change a wet top were more frequent in my first 5 years of practice. Focussing our practice where possible to maximise our experience certainly reduces stress levels. Having a senior mentor in the early years is also a big help.

Ensuring the whole team is forewarned and aware of potential problems is an important safety net. The morning 'briefing' where the surgery list is discussed, followed by a thorough 'time out' before each case, ensures each member is tuned to potential problems.

When things inevitably do go wrong, I suggest

- Stop/pause/think.
- Three deep breaths.
- Respectfully and honestly communicate the problem to your team.
- Outline the options and choose your best way forward.
- Ask the opinion of a colleague (even through a phone call).
- Ask the opinion of your team.
  - Two years ago, I experienced the heart-stopping complication of a significant popliteal artery injury during a difficult HTO. A senior scrub nurse knew that my vascular surgeon colleague was just down the road getting his car serviced! A life (and limb) saver.
- Keep your hands soft on the instruments.
- Seek help quickly when required (see above).

When a member of our team makes an error

- Stop (take three breaths if required).
- Respectfully explain why it is an error and how to avoid it in the future.
- Increase communication. Always take time to explain WHY we are doing it this way rather than demanding a series of meaningless steps. (I have heard surgeons answer an intelligent question from a scrub nurse with "You do not need to know.")
- Maintain all staff member's dignity. Their aspirations for the patient's wellbeing are similar to yours.
- Our operating room teams love hearing how our patients are doing, seeing pictures of their accomplishments and reading emails of their latest adventure. An investment in what we are doing results in everyone in the room giving their best.

It was Franklin D. Roosevelt who said "We have nothing to fear but fear itself." It is worth thinking about what we are afraid of. A poor patient outcome? Loss of reputation? Loss of respect from colleagues? All of the above? Self-awareness is often the first step towards positive change. The angry shouting surgeon is not giving their best to their team or themselves. The most important person is anaesthetised under the drapes and not in a position to change their mind and walk out on poor behaviour.

The End of Sports Surgery

Andrew A. Amis

While the ISAKOS congress always includes many technical papers about the minutiae of surgical techniques, and we strive to develop the procedures, which will lead to the best outcomes following sports injuries, these concerns pale into insignificance in relation to the looming possibility that the entire field may be wiped out in the foreseeable future, so that the sports surgeon may become extinct. What may cause such a catastrophe for the field? I believe, based on an increasing level of reports in the press, that routine surgery may become more hazardous with the proliferation of antibiotic-resistant microorganisms. It is being suggested that what are now routine surgeries such as joint replacement arthroplasty may cease because of the possibility of untreatable infections.

Although there is increasing realisation of the dangers resulting from indiscriminate use of antibiotics in the more highly developed countries, there are many ways in which the situation may continue to become uncontrollable, and thus, the misuse of antibiotics spreads further across the world. The press includes stories such as the sale of what may or may not be genuine drugs through the Internet and of those who have nonbacterial infections demanding antibiotics from their doctors, or else acquiring them elsewhere and then not taking the correct treatment course. Clearly, there is much to be done on this front for educating people.

Farming is a culprit in the indiscriminate use of antibiotics because there are efficiency gains to be made from pre-emptive dosing of entire herds of animals. This can be to promote growth rather than to fight infection, so farmers are incentivised to ignore rules that try to limit the use of antibiotics when, perhaps, they could use inoculation to prevent herds being vulnerable to specific diseases. Agricultural use is leading to increasing levels of antibiotics present in the run-off from farms (along, also, with other chemicals such as nitrates from fertiliser). The more immediate

A. A. Amis (✉)
The Biomechanics Group, Department of Mechanical Engineering,
Imperial College London, London, UK
e-mail: a.amis@imperial.ac.uk

© ISAKOS 2020
B. M. Devitt et al. (eds.), *The Future of Orthopaedic Sports Medicine*,
https://doi.org/10.1007/978-3-030-28976-8_21

problem for us is that indiscriminate agricultural use provides more opportunities for the microorganisms to develop antibiotic resistance, and the farmers are often using the same antibiotics as are used in human clinical work.

A worrying factor is the frequency of air travel these days, so that infected people can spread antibiotic-resistant organisms internationally almost before serious problems are recognised. And then where are we treated for these infections? In a hospital, a place where there are many patients who are carrying their own sets of infectious microorganisms, an ideal scenario for breeding antibiotic resistance or encountering resistant microorganisms.

The WHO reports that 'antibiotic resistance is rising to dangerously high levels in all parts of the world' and that infections such as pneumonia and tuberculosis are becoming harder or sometimes impossible to treat. They note that antibiotic resistance is emerging and spreading worse in countries without standard treatment guidelines, with over-prescription by health workers and veterinarians, and over-use by the anxious public. Meanwhile, there is increasing difficulty in discovering new antibiotics of last resort. It seems that efforts to halt this worrying trend should include many stakeholders, from health carers taking on greater thoroughness in infection control, the public also doing so and being educated about correct use of a course of antibiotics and the limitations of them to treat non-bacterial infections, and agriculture becoming more discriminating and/or regulated. In the meantime, those who treat these resistant infections must harbour their ammunition carefully, and maybe the pharma industry and healthcare regulators must get together to try to prevent the leakage of the antibiotics of last resort into the wider realm. There has been much publicity about this topic in the UK recently, following a warning call for action from the government's Chief Medical Officer, but there is not much evidence of it being a priority for politicians.

If the present trend is not halted, and a whole new class of antimicrobials is not suddenly discovered, it appears that surgery on vulnerable patients such as in organ transplantation may become very high risk. In that scenario, maybe sports injuries and their related surgery will become more feared, as the likelihood of an untreatable infection following even a superficial injury becomes widely known, while the possibility of untreatable infection during surgery causes many patients to decide to live with their disability, rather than face that danger. So I am worried that, one day not so far in the future, we shall enter a post-surgery era, when ISAKOS, sports surgeons, their arthroscopes and interference screws may only be found in history books…

Will Our Focus on Techniques and Technology to Improve Patient Outcomes Be at the Expense of a Loss of Clinical Judgement?

Julian A. Feller

Robotics is making its mark in joint replacement and gaining in popularity. Whether it improves patient outcomes in the longer term remains to be seen. After all, despite the enthusiastic use of robotics for prostatectomy for more than a decade, the evidence to show improved outcomes is thin on the ground. But surgeons have a natural tendency to explore technology that might facilitate a surgical procedure or–and this is perhaps sceptical and even unkind–improve their profile and attract patients.

Robotic drilling of femoral and tibial tunnels for anterior cruciate ligament (ACL) reconstruction is a real possibility. But will it improve outcomes? Who knows? For all the research and innovation in ACL reconstruction over the past 25 years, our results have not dramatically improved. The 'ideal' bone tunnel positions have changed over time but with little change in clinical outcomes. Will 'augmented reality' and robots alter this? Certainly, one can envisage more reliable placement of the tunnel where we think it should be but knowing where it should be is the first step. As for all developments and research, we should always start with a simple question; what is the problem we want to solve? With regard to tunnel position in ACL reconstruction, that question is probably one of where rather than of how.

Similarly, there is an assumption that better restoration of anatomy will improve outcomes. New instrumentation facilitates repair of posterior root tears of the lateral meniscus, repair of ramp lesions of the posterior horn of the medial meniscus and repair or reconstruction of injuries to the anterolateral complex. Whilst these structures all undoubtedly contribute to the stability of the ACL-injured knee, does their repair really restore anatomy and improve outcomes? Time zero laboratory studies on cadaveric specimens may produce encouraging graphs, but it is a significant leap of faith to assume that there will be a

J. A. Feller (✉)
OrthoSport Victoria, Melbourne, VIC, Australia
e-mail: jfeller@osv.com.au

© ISAKOS 2020
B. M. Devitt et al. (eds.), *The Future of Orthopaedic Sports Medicine*,
https://doi.org/10.1007/978-3-030-28976-8_22

concomitant improvement in clinical outcomes. Yet, we are nonetheless drawn to the technical possibilities and the opportunity to develop new procedures and instrumentation.

Artificial intelligence is a powerful tool that can analyse the results of blood tests and see trends that predict a deterioration in a patient's status well before we humans can. Or analyse imaging or an ECG with greater accuracy and reliability than a human. Presumably, artificial intelligence will be or is already able to analyse a patient's responses to a series of questions–the history!–as well as their imaging and provide a diagnosis with an accuracy on par with a good clinician.

Does getting the diagnosis right and performing technically excellent surgery lead to better results? One hopes and even presumes that they contribute to a better outcome. But there is a fundamental step between making a diagnosis and performing surgery that is probably at least as important, if not more important, than either the diagnosis or skilful surgery–selecting the appropriate intervention for the individual patient.

That intervention may well be non-surgical. We have heard much in recent years about the role of arthroscopy in the treatment of medial meniscal tears. There are some who interpret the 'evidence' as indicating there is little or no role for arthroscopy anymore. I sometimes wonder whether knee arthroscopy would have gained popularity as fast as it did if there were no medial meniscus, for it was the dramatic improvement in recovery from medial meniscectomy that really highlighted the benefits of this surgical tool. But have we over-used the tool just because it makes for a minimally invasive and usually low-morbidity procedure? Has the apparent simplicity of the procedure clouded our judgement about when to use it?

So many of the studies in this area have failed to clarify whether failure of non-operative management of a medial meniscal tear was a requirement for consideration of arthroscopic intervention, let alone describe the relevant clinical findings–apart from reporting 'mechanical symptoms', at best a somewhat nebulous phrase that is harder to define than it first appears. Even if strict objective indications for surgical intervention are used, experience–the basis of clinical judgement– should help us predict when arthroscopic intervention is likely to help and, far more importantly, when it is not likely to help and should therefore be avoided.

Evidence-based practice does not really emphasise a role for clinical judgement, other than to assume that good clinical judgement has been exercised. We are now bombarded through social media with 'evidence' for a particular course of intervention, whether that evidence stands up to scrutiny or not. Two hundred and eighty characters do not allow for a detailed analysis. Yet, by sheer weight of the number of times, it is re-circulated, a simple statement or proposition can acquire an authority greater than it deserves. Skilful use of social media allows individuals to rapidly reach a large audience and potentially change thinking and practice. Our increasingly 'digital' way of thinking does not encourage measured consideration–the application of clinical judgement.

My worry is that orthopaedic surgeons will be seduced by techniques and technology and forget that the best way to achieve a good outcome from surgery is to do the right operation on the right patient at the right time in the natural history of their problem.

Don Johnson

When I first started orthopedic practice in 1973, an ACL injury was career ending. We did not really know how to diagnose the injury and certainly had no idea of what to do even if it was diagnosed at open surgery when performing a meniscectomy. But just how did the evolution of ACL surgery occur?

Advances were slow in the 1970s and 1980s. David MacIntosh taught us how to diagnose the ACL-deficient knee with his pivot shift description and how to perform an extra-articular reconstruction, which eventually evolved to the intra-articular quadriceps patella tendon graft placed in the top position. This was later refined to the free patella tendon graft by Erickson and Bill. You had to be a real athlete to survive these big open operations, and consequently, the recreational athlete was treated conservatively. The Marshall primary repair was initially popular but fell into disrepute after a high failure rate was reported.

The four-bundle hamstring graft came into popular use in the late 1980s and 1990s. We had a limited choice of guides to place the tunnels, but the rear entry guide did a very good job of placing the femoral tunnel in the correct position. The single incision transtibial guide was introduced in 1995 and became popular even though the tunnel position was high in the notch.

During this time, we were more concerned about the technique but not so much about the results and particularly the rates of return to sport. The international knee documentation committee (IKDC) scale helped a lot in the objective measurements of outcome, but we were still not eliminating the pivot shift. We felt that the return to sport was good in elite athletes, but when we started to look more closely at results in others, it was disappointing. Julian Feller showed <50% return to sports with the quadruple hamstring grafts in high-level athletes. It was also reported that there was a 20% failure of hamstring grafts in the adolescent patient group. Allografts in the young population had similarly poor results. The patient-reported

D. Johnson (✉)
Department of Orthopaedics, University of Ottawa, Ottawa, ON, Canada
e-mail: johnson_don@me.com

© ISAKOS 2020
B. M. Devitt et al. (eds.), *The Future of Orthopaedic Sports Medicine*,
https://doi.org/10.1007/978-3-030-28976-8_23

outcomes were also less than optimum. We also hadn't recognized that many patients did not return to the same sport, same position, and the same level. Some of the reasons it transpired related to the fear of re-injury. Rehabilitation had focused on the physical recuperation but not on mental recovery. Admittedly, elite athletes have had a better return to sports rate.

So, should we be worried? Of course, it seems that after 40 years, we have several options for graft choice in ACL reconstructions that have not changed over the past 20 years. The failure rate, return to sport at the same level, same position, and the same sport has not really improved. I am sure some of the younger physicians are going to look back on these procedures such as '*ripping out your hamstrings*' as barbaric. Let's take off the rose-colored glasses and realize that we are not as good as we think we are, or how good we tell the patient they are going to be after surgery.

23.1   Where Should We Look for Improvement?

Firstly, does everyone need an ACL reconstruction? Maybe some more folks should be encouraged to change activities to avoid pivotal sports. This should also be an option after the operation. The biological enhancement of primary ACL repair may be one area that I think has great promise. Biologics in general are going to be an expensive option that our medical system may not be able to afford. The primary repair is really only an option in a small sub-group of patients, usually proximal tears in skiers. Most of the tears in soccer, basketball, and football are mid-substance tears not amenable to this option.

23.2   What We Should Be Worried About?

In the first 20 years, we made significant advances in diagnosis with Lachman and pivot shift tests, imaging, and choice of graft. In the second 20 years, we have tweaked the technique, keep the same graft choice (robbing Peter to pay Paul concept) but have not significantly improved the objective stability, failure rate, or return to sport rate.

Please Take Your Time: A Research Perspective

24

Kate E. Webster

As a PhD student midway through my candidature, I distinctly recall my supervisor telling me to take my time and read as widely as I could, because from this point forward, my life would only become busier. He explained that soon I would no longer have the luxury of time to indulge my learning in the same way that was currently possible. I can't recall how I responded but remember shaking my head as I walked away thinking that I was already really busy! Fast forward 20 years and I now find myself giving the exact same advice to my own students. I am sure they don't entirely believe my words, as I didn't when the same advice was given to me, but I persist anyway for a number of reasons, which I expand upon below.

The first reason is learning the fundamentals. I am concerned that my students, and many others, aren't investing the time to understand the basics of good scientific research. They are in too much of a hurry, and this is in part a symptom of the world in which we now live. I urge students, and anyone undertaking research, to take the time to learn all they can about methodological design, as this underpins all good scientific research. I urge them to take those extra statistics courses too, and I assure them that they will come in handy! They need to be able to understand their data. They need to emerge themselves in the research culture and learn all they can from as many people as they can.

The second reason, which overlaps with the first, is related to the ability to scrutinize scientific evidence. On a daily basis, we are literally bombarded with information, and the information is so readily available. Too often, we see Twitter and other forms of media as a sole source of information gathering. Whilst such sources are beneficial for awareness, they do not replace reading and fully scrutinizing a research paper. I can unequivocally state that in my student days, there was not one research paper that I didn't fully read if I had taken the effort and time and monetary investment to go to the library (which I had to do), locate the journal and paid the

K. E. Webster (✉)
School of Allied Health, La Trobe University, Melbourne, VIC, Australia
e-mail: K.Webster@latrobe.edu.au

© ISAKOS 2020
B. M. Devitt et al. (eds.), *The Future of Orthopaedic Sports Medicine*,
https://doi.org/10.1007/978-3-030-28976-8_24

photocopy fee. We virtually never go to the library anymore because we can download everything we need, usually for free. I therefore see piles of unread articles on both mine and my student's desks. We fall into the fallacy that we have done the work by simply printing the paper and reading the abstract. Too often, we rely on the authors' conclusions. This is not good enough, and we must always question the methods and the conclusions of all scientific research, and then form our own judgements. Consider all the evidence, not just the loudest voice.

Beyond the academic contribution, we also need to consider the impact our research makes in terms of its contribution to the economy, society, culture or environment. Metrics are important for a number of reasons but they are not everything. Our primary outcome should be asking the most relevant questions and conducting the best possible research we can. Take research seriously but also love it and have fun doing it, as that is what makes it all worthwhile to both the scientist and their audience!

What's in It for Me?

25

Thomas P. Branch

As orthopedic sports medicine specialists, we need to "treat patients, who need to be treated, and not treat patients, who do not need to be treated." If we don't abide by this moniker, we may price ourselves out of business as it is today. In fact, we are headed there already.

The number of new and innovative treatment options in orthopedic sports medicine has multiplied over my lifetime. No longer do we need to filet patients open to fix torn or broken parts; we have the arthroscope and minimally invasive surgery. With the tools that have been invented, sports medicine physicians can fix just about anything given the opportunity. What worries me is the question of when should we treat. Is there really a surgical or biological fix for every patient complaint? What happened to activity modification and a structured exercise program? Or at least some treatment that is less expensive to society?

We continue to operate at an alarming rate. When I started as a resident, a patient with an anterior cruciate-deficient knee was categorized into three groups: those who could not cope with their ACL-deficient knee and thus needed reconstructive surgery, those who could easily cope with an ACL-deficient knee under any condition and did not need surgery, and those who could cope with the ligament deficiency with significant activity modification and only might need surgery. In today's world, if a patient with an ACL-deficient knee passes within 100 m of a sports medicine surgeon, they receive one and sometimes two reconstructions.

In my generation, we learned that a 3 mm side-to-side difference in a standard Lachman test indicates anterior cruciate ligament deficiency. Post-ACL reconstructed patients looking for relief of symptoms travel from one orthopedic surgeon to the next. Oftentimes, they find themselves with a second ligament reconstruction if there is any increased anterior play in their knee. Yet, when revision ACL surgery is evaluated, there is a markedly diminished success rate. Why? Perhaps repeating the same procedure that failed will not address the patient's problem. Recently, I

T. P. Branch (✉)
University Orthopedics, Atlanta, GA, USA

© ISAKOS 2020
B. M. Devitt et al. (eds.), *The Future of Orthopaedic Sports Medicine*,
https://doi.org/10.1007/978-3-030-28976-8_25

have had to arthroscopically remove ACL reconstructions in knees that are biomechanically too tight. These patients were relieved to have a more normal feeling knee. In these instances, ACL reconstruction was simply not the right thing to do.

If orthopedic sports medicine surgeons continue to operate at their current rate, what will happen? The social cost of medicine is a major portion of a country's gross national product. In the United States, we are already seeing insurance companies using every potential tactic to delay or obfuscate surgeons in their quest to approve a surgical intervention. Driven by economics, the choices available to us and, ultimately, our patients will soon go away. Protocols and algorithms will be constructed by healthcare specialists with public health degrees who use obscure research for justification. Relegated to "technician status," orthopedic sports medicine surgeons will need to be told what to do for their patients.

The following question begs to be raised: How can I do my part to reduce health care costs? The surgeon must learn to choose treatment plans wisely. The inactive patient doesn't need a new ACL. The athlete needs time off with a detailed home exercise program rather than a scope followed by the same. The tennis player needs coaching instructions and core training instead of a repeat acromioplasty. It is time for us to be the solution for rising healthcare costs and not the cause.

What is in it for me? The answer is freedom to practice the art of medicine.

Social Media in Sports Medicine

Mihai Vioreanu

> *The secret of change is to focus all of your energy, not on fighting the old, but on building the new.*
>
> —Socrates

Whether we like or not, the fast growth of social media is having a major impact on our personal and professional lives.

Social media is the space where patients are engaging, sharing their healthcare experiences and seeking health information. More people than ever are searching online for health information. In 2009, PEW research in the USA reported that 61% of adult Internet users had looked online for health information [1]. By 2014, that number had grown to 72% [2]. According to a recent PEW research in the USA, at least 80% of Americans are turning to Dr. Google before an actual doctor. Among patients presenting to an orthopaedic academic centre in the USA, sports medicine patients were found to be the highest users of social media [3].

Healthcare professionals find their own value in online health information. Ninety per cent of physicians consider the internet to be an indispensable professional resource, relying heavily on it for immediately accessible guidance. Following what their peers are discussing and sharing is the most popular social media activity for 60% of physicians [4]. Video platforms such as Vumedi, where surgeons share surgical techniques and debate specialised topics in the field of orthopaedic and sports medicine surgery, are becoming increasingly popular among surgeons. For these physicians, a significant part of their professional life and networking has moved online. More and more healthcare professionals are using social media platforms such as LinkedIn for searching jobs [4].

M. Vioreanu (✉)
Sports Surgery Clinic, Dublin, Ireland
e-mail: mihai@mihaivioreanu.com

© ISAKOS 2020

B. M. Devitt et al. (eds.), *The Future of Orthopaedic Sports Medicine*,
https://doi.org/10.1007/978-3-030-28976-8_26

There are many benefits for both the healthcare consumer and the healthcare provider from engaging on social media. Social media helps to educate patients and build awareness of available care and treatments for their condition. Social media helps the healthcare consumer to engage with fellow patients and share their healthcare experiences and results of their treatments. Social media can build a sense of community among patients. Equally, social media offers a two-way conduit through which healthcare providers (i.e., surgeon, physician, physiotherapist, etc.) and their patients can interact. Various social media platforms provide us with an audience of patients, many of whom are already organised in patient groups that are actively seeking information and interaction with professionals. Social media can help the patients trust us more. Building trust in healthcare is vital and sometimes can be a challenge. Empathetic behaviour is one of the best ways to build trust, and social media can be a great tool for expressing and sharing empathy. Social media helps us gauge the patients' expectations and satisfaction with our services. It is an easy place to gather feedback and to get a sense of how satisfied the patient is with you. Social media lets you tell your story. It's a way for the patient to learn not only what you do but also why you do it and what your values are. Social media tends to be a more cost-effective method in engaging with the healthcare consumer than the traditional advertising by allowing us to address a specific audience more easily and directly. Essentially, social media in healthcare, when used properly, can result in an efficient and effective means of communicating with our patients.

At the same time, social media can also have a negative impact on patients' healthcare experience. This potential deleterious effect makes me worried about the use of social media by healthcare providers when used without ethical consideration. The concern is that 'fake news' in healthcare is rampant, so when patients reach for health information online, they may find information that is untrue and potentially dangerous. Often this information contributes to patients developing unrealistic expectations and lures them in with the prospect of 'miracle cures'. Also, there is a tendency by patients to share this information widely in an act of altruism to let others in on the great secret. In turn, building unrealistic expectations will lead to patient disappointment. If something sounds too good to be true, the reason typically is because it is not true! More often than not, the 'miracle cure', which is claimed to be 'scientifically proven', is not supported by rigorous scientific evidence. What is worse, when the treatment fails, it is not just the patient who suffers but the whole medical profession, as the trust and faith that we have spent centuries developing are quickly eroded.

In order to promote the benefits of social media engagement in sports medicine and at the same time protect our patients from its potential negative impact, we should be aware of the potential pitfalls and risk of social media and be careful when using this tool to disseminate and promote healthcare knowledge and research findings. As patients' advocates, sports medicine clinicians should actively engage in social media for the benefit of both their patients and their practices, but we should do it carefully and respectfully with ethical and scientific rigour.

References

1. Fox S. Online health search 2006 (Pew Internet Project: October 29, 2006). http://www.pewinternet.org/Reports/2006/Online-Health-Search-2006.aspx.
2. http://www.pewresearch.org/fact-tank/2014/01/15/the-social-life-of-health-information/.
3. Curry E, Li X, Nguyen J, Matzkin E. Prevalence of internet and social media usage in orthopedic surgery. Orthop Rev. 2014;6(3):5483.
4. http://www.cdwcommunit.com/resources/infographic/social-media/.

Biologic and Regenerative Medicine: The Balance Between Promise and Proven

27

Jason L. Koh

In many ways, the future of sports medicine is extremely bright. We are living in a day and age when we continue to discover new knowledge and innovative new treatments are being developed to treat sports injuries. Our understanding of the human body and sports medicine injuries has never been greater, and new biologic and regenerative techniques hold the promise of being able to restore function in ways never before dreamed possible. However, the challenge lies in balancing the possible with the proven in the treatment of patients.

There is enormous interest in using biological and regenerative treatments to harness the body's own abilities to heal and regrow tissue to help address degeneration and trauma. The excitement generated by these concepts has spread into the popular media. Newspaper advertisements sell stem cell treatments for arthritis; the television announces that professional athletes are injecting plasma, growth factors, or hormones. Clinics and companies have sprung up selling amniotic membranes and nasal cell transplants and other tissues and treatments that have very little assessment or evaluation. Patients eagerly seek these solutions and spend millions of dollars, when, in many cases, excellent treatments (both operative and nonoperative) exist. Meanwhile, researchers struggle to get support to perform the critical studies needed to assess the value of these new therapies.

There is a concerning dichotomy between the popular perception of what these treatments can accomplish, and the actual results from research studies. There is strong evidence from well-done studies that some biologic and regenerative treatments can help alleviate pain and restore function; there are also studies that do not demonstrate any significant differences between certain treatments and active controls or placebos. Where the challenge for sports medicine arises is continuing to perform the difficult work of good evidence-based medicine, while trying to address the immediate needs of the injured athlete. Patients come and demand treatments, or

J. L. Koh (✉)
Mark R. Neaman Family Chair of Orthopaedic Surgery, NorthShore Orthopaedic and Spine Institute, Evanston, IL, USA

© ISAKOS 2020
B. M. Devitt et al. (eds.), *The Future of Orthopaedic Sports Medicine*,
https://doi.org/10.1007/978-3-030-28976-8_27

there may be time pressure to accelerate healing or recovery, particularly in a sports-related situation where there may be a limited season or critical game. In some situations, other therapeutic options may have already been tried and exhausted. In these circumstances, the treating clinician may consider making a choice to try a new therapy that may have limited data that support its use. The risk exists that unnecessary or ineffective treatments may be performed, to the detriment of the patient.

We must continue to explore and learn more to improve our treatments. Biologic and regenerative medicine treatments are likely to be an integral part of our therapeutic armamentarium in the future, but their precise role and function remain to be determined. They are not likely to be a panacea that can cure all ills; rather, we must critically evaluate the evidence and clearly communicate what the data show. Continued thoughtful research will be critical for our ability to understand the true value of these therapies. In this way, we can work together to best inform and treat our sports medicine patients.

There Are No Facts, Only Interpretations

28

John M. O'Byrne

My concerns with regard to sports medicine and its future is the discrepancy between the sophistication and quality and detail of the investigations available to us, and their interpretation. The investigations can be sub divided into two broad categories: those that study structure, which are sophisticated imaging techniques, and those that study function, which are very elaborate performance assessment tools.

My first experience of disappointment at the weak link that can exist between sophisticated measurement and clinical relevance occurred in the early 1990s, when, as an orthopaedic resident, I carried out a Masters in Surgery thesis research under the supervision of the late and iconic Professor Tim O'Brien. The aim of the thesis was to analyse the massive amount of raw data that were generated in a gait laboratory, looking at kinematic patterns of walking in children with cerebral palsy and try and identify clinical sub-types and treatment protocols. The assessment technology was, for that time, very sophisticated and generated huge volumes of very accurate measurement data.

Using cluster statistics on these numerical values, we sub-divided the gait patterns into different types. We then endeavoured to identify clinical characteristics of each of these sub-types. It was a very clunky and crude and forced way of picking clinical patterns and pathologies out of large amounts of raw data using a form of artificial intelligence.

However, I believe it was laudable in its attempts to close the gap between sophisticated methods of measurement and its interpretation for a clinician, using automatic data analysis.

In the context of sports medicine, there is a dizzying array of measurements of performance activity and movement. Many of these measurements no longer require laboratory analysis but are based on a smartphone or a bracelet.

J. M. O'Byrne (✉)
Royal College of Surgeons in Ireland, Dublin, Ireland
e-mail: jmobyrne@rcsi.ie

© ISAKOS 2020
B. M. Devitt et al. (eds.), *The Future of Orthopaedic Sports Medicine*,
https://doi.org/10.1007/978-3-030-28976-8_28

When I read about these data, I study very carefully the evidence that links the quality and sophistication of the data gathering with the clinical conclusions and recommendations. I must confess at many times I have that feeling I originally had with the gait analysis data that the interpretation and understanding of what it means is massively behind the quality or presentation of the data. It is easy to be seduced and dazzled by the quality of technology making the measurement and not carefully study the clinical conclusions or recommendations that are being made.

With regard to structure, as orthopaedic surgeons, we are the first and foremost students of anatomy. It is therefore very exciting to experience new and sophisticated imaging modalities. Technology has advanced at such a rate that one can almost microscopically examine the musculoskeletal system using modern MR techniques. However, again, the interpretation and appearances and understanding of what is normal and abnormal lags behind the quality of patient measurements. It is also worth noting that in many areas of orthopaedic surgery, our objective assessments of the patients' function and our imaging of their structure have disappointingly not always correlated with patient-reported outcomes. In other words, the patients just don't seem to appreciate how good looking the X-ray is!

Sports medicine is a very exciting field with increasing use of technology to assess and improve functions. This applies not only purely in terms of the sports medicine aspect of the modern game but also in terms of player performance assessment. However, the point is made regularly, that the player with very good statistics in terms of speed, distance covered and pass completion, may not necessarily have had a 'good game' or 'changed the game and driven on the team'.

There will always be a need to combine a holistic impression with sophisticated and detailed measurements.

Like all orthopaedic surgeons, I embrace and welcome new and sophisticated technology. However, I do occasionally have that nagging feeling that the data are somehow being forced into a clinical meaning or implication, in some instances, to justify the highly sophisticated technology. Technology to assess structure and function is fantastic, but its interpretation and clinical implications must be carefully studied.

Oh, and by the way, some of those children with cerebral palsy that we studied had the most abnormal kinematic patterns…….. but, boy, could they move!!

Increased Incidence of Sports Trauma in Children. Is It Time to Worry?

29

Vojtech Havlas

In our clinical practice, we are confronted with an increasing number of paediatric trauma due to sporting injuries. In the past decade, the number of children treated for joint and musculoskeletal pathology has increased dramatically. Although surgical techniques in sports medicine are rapidly evolving and we have a wide range of treatment options in our arsenal, we are facing more challenging cases in younger patients.

In the past, paediatric trauma mostly relied on conservative treatment. Although the healing potential of young individual is very strong and it is helping us significantly in our efforts, it has its limitations. Surgical treatment becomes a treatment option more often than in the past. Not only the incidence of sports trauma increases, but also the severity of children's trauma is worsening. In paediatric traumatology, we are facing types of trauma that were typical for adult patients in the past, such as complex knee ligament injuries, severe cartilage defects or comminuted fractures. Despite our efforts to minimise the impact of these trauma and the healing potential of children's body, it is imminent that, in the future, we will have to face the sequelae. We have to bear in mind that every trauma and surgical procedure leaves permanent changes in anatomy and physiology of the body.

For example, in the field of knee surgery and ligament reconstruction, we more and more often treat patients at the age of 10–15 years (and even younger) with complete ACL ruptures. Despite the use of modern techniques to reconstruct ligaments without the risk of growth plate damage resulting in growth deterioration, the number of failed surgeries or recurrent trauma is increasing in our patient cohort. We might say that the younger the patient at the time of surgery, the higher is the chance to recurrent trauma or failed surgery. Do we have enough safe and proven techniques to treat these cases?

V. Havlas (✉)
Department of Orthopaedics and Traumatology, 2nd Faculty of Medicine,
Charles University in Prague, Prague, Czech Republic

© ISAKOS 2020   75
B. M. Devitt et al. (eds.), *The Future of Orthopaedic Sports Medicine*,
https://doi.org/10.1007/978-3-030-28976-8_29

Even more challenging are severe cartilage defects in adolescents. The number of children that are indicated for surgical treatment of large osteochondral defect is growing constantly. We have a wide range of surgical techniques to reconstruct cartilage; however, the results are not always fully satisfactory. On the contrary, significantly more patients are presenting with severe joint degeneration due to sports trauma in the young patient group under 30 years of age. Are we ready to treat these patients? In the future, the economical impact of this trend might become a severe problem.

We might ask: What is the reason for this increase in sports trauma? Is it the fact that professional sport is attracting a larger number of children and parents, or is the children's population having problems with musculoskeletal coordination? Is there any way to reduce the negative trend in increasing of paediatric trauma? One would say we need more specialised centres to treat these difficult and challenging cases and more skilled and experienced surgeons to treat our young patients. Or is there not a time to improve cooperation with authorities and sports clubs in the field of prevention? All surgeons treating children should ask these questions and make an effort to support the prevention programmes. Unless we stop this negative trend of increase in paediatric trauma and its consequences, it is time to start worrying about our future.

Persistent Lack of Patient Treatment Outcome Information for Patients, Therapists, and Surgeons

Marc Swiontkowski

Orthopedic surgery was the first surgical specialty to engage in a broad spread initiative to understand patient-oriented outcomes. In 1990, Clement Sledge, MD, in his role in the AAOS presidential line, established an outcomes committee. This effort was, in large part, informed by the seminal work of Dr. John Wennberg at Dartmouth. The research approach of small area analysis, developed by Dr. Wennberg, was fairly early on applied to the musculoskeletal system as one of the most common clinical scenarios requiring or resulting in invasive interventions. He established that residents of the postal codes around Boston were four times more likely to undergo hip replacement than residents of the area around New Haven, Connecticut, and residents of those postal codes were four times more likely to undergo a spinal procedure than residents of Boston. He identified that one major impact in these discrepancies, besides local surgeon culture and density, was the lack of information on what outcomes of importance patients could expect to experience. The AAOS embarked on a program called MODEMS with the goal of encouraging surgeons to measure their patient-oriented outcomes—functional outcomes rather than simply the clinical outcomes (infection, range of motion, and strength) that we typically measured. Several patient-oriented measures were developed and validated, but the program was abandoned after 3 years due to the high cost of investment with little promise of financial return from the program.

The academic orthopedic community persisted with investments in developing and validating patient-reported outcome measures (PROMs) and incorporating the use of these tools to accompany standard clinical outcomes as a regular part of reporting trial results in peer-reviewed journals. However, the efforts to have the processes of collecting relevant patient outcomes by the "rank and file" have never recovered. Those individuals and practices that participated in the MODEMS

M. Swiontkowski (✉)
Department of Orthopaedic Surgery, University of Minnesota, Minneapolis, MN, USA

TRIA Orthopaedic Center, Bloomington, MN, USA
e-mail: swion001@umn.edu

© ISAKOS 2020   77
B. M. Devitt et al. (eds.), *The Future of Orthopaedic Sports Medicine*,
https://doi.org/10.1007/978-3-030-28976-8_30

program discovered that they had data, lots of data. However, the data were collected from patients with numerous interventions and numerous timeframes and were not organized in a way that analyses could be completed in a manner that resulted in meaningful information to be shared with patients in order to inform their decision-making regarding indications, risks and benefits for treatment options being discussed by their surgeon or therapist. Members of the community of sports surgeons, physicians, and therapists participated along the same lines with other academically oriented surgeons developing and validating functional outcomes and activity scales that were applied to contributions to the peer-review literature. In a similar way, widespread use of these tools outside of the research environment is largely absent.

How then do therapists, physicians, and surgeons provide information on expected outcomes to patients considering treatment options in the area of sports medicine? The answer is in the same way that practitioners in other subspecialties do; they quote the peer-reviewed literature to their patients. Practitioners generally have no idea how their patients are doing with regard to clinical and functional outcomes without a systematic approach to explaining to patients why we need this information and how they, the patient, can contribute to improving the results for others with similar injuries or disorders. Often our treatment recommendations are based on what we learned in residency or fellowship without any sort of review of patient outcome data. Perhaps worse, they are based on one or two terrible results or two to three outstanding results, which form an overall impression of the success of an intervention. It is well known in research, which focuses on patient outcomes, as it relates to volumes of interventions, that higher volumes generally result in overall improved outcomes. This is true for any sort of complex intervention, including surgical procedures or rehabilitation protocols. A surgeon who performs 20 ACL reconstructions simply cannot reliably quote the results of the MOON group to their patients. They could be better but in all likelihood are probably not as good. The only way to offer patients accurate information on their potential challenges and upside to a particular treatment is to measure our own outcomes and consistently analyze and report those results to our patients and their families.

What really worries me is that the incentives to engage in this activity remain lacking as they have ever since the demise of our initial attempts in the 1990s. Efforts have been focused on tools to collect this information—software, touch screens, remote sensors, etc. Tools do not create the incentives and may, by their expense and steep learning curves, produce a negative effect. Patients do not have incentives to provide us this information once they are outside the active treatment period. None of us, neither patients nor providers, likes to complete surveys of any sort and physician requests to respond to validated surveys are no different. Establishing systems to follow patients and get the PROM data at select times from graduation from a rehabilitation program or post-surgical treatment are expensive in terms of personnel and physician time.

I can foresee a time when patients can be incentivized by their insurance carrier to provide this information by lower premiums or co-pays. I can foresee a time when insurers pay physician, therapist, and surgeon providers a higher rate to compensate for this activity. What really worries me is that I have seen almost no action in these areas. Patients and insurers are content with physicians, therapists, and surgeons, offering them outcome data from very high-volume expert providers as if these were from the providers who will be providing the care. Persistence of this situation should scare everyone involved. It is like deciding on car safety with no crash test performance data. None of us would participate in such reckless behavior, yet we allow the current system to persist when quality of life and limb function are truly at risk.

The Perils and Potentials of Biologic Therapies

31

Scott Rodeo

I believe that one of the challenges faced in the field of musculoskeletal surgery is the great potential but also pitfalls of "biologic" approaches for augmentation of tissue healing. There is universal agreement that cytokines, novel small peptides, platelet-rich plasma, and other blood-derived products, stem cells, innovative biomaterials, and gene therapy techniques all hold tremendous promise for improvement in healing of many types of musculoskeletal tissues. However, there are currently a number of scientific, logistical, and regulatory hurdles to overcome before these therapies can be used on a widespread basis.

The area of cell-based therapies for improvement of tissue healing provides a good example of the numerous outstanding issues that need to be resolved. The currently available options include cells derived from bone marrow and adipose tissue. However, the number of true stem cells by formal molecular criteria is very small in these tissues. Thus, optimal use of these approaches requires ex vivo cell sorting and culture expansion. Such cell manipulation is costly, and there are still unanswered questions about the optimal cell culturing protocols to identify and maintain pluripotent cells. Furthermore, the regulatory environment varies between different countries. For example, in the USA, ex vivo "manipulation" (culture expansion) of bone marrow or adipose tissue samples is not allowed.

Even once we do obtain a large number of purified stem cells, there are further significant biologic challenges. It is well established that cells may change their phenotype once dissociated from their native environment. Transplantation to a new

S. Rodeo (✉)
Sports Medicine and Shoulder Service, New York, NY, USA

Orthopaedic Soft Tissue Research Program, New York, NY, USA

Orthopaedic Surgery, Weill Medical College of Cornell University, New York, NY, USA

The Hospital for Special Surgery, New York, NY, USA

New York Giants Football, New York, NY, USA
e-mail: RodeoS@HSS.EDU

© ISAKOS 2020
B. M. Devitt et al. (eds.), *The Future of Orthopaedic Sports Medicine*,
https://doi.org/10.1007/978-3-030-28976-8_31

environment with different nutritional and oxidative requirements will further affect the biology and activity of the cells. Further information is required to identify the optimal signals that are required to stimulate the cells for optimal function. Extensive further research is required to define the appropriate soluble cues to stimulate transplanted cells. Defining these signals requires identification of the biologic target that we are trying to treat: Is the goal to increase cell proliferation in the new tissue? Stimulate matrix synthesis? Increase angiogenesis? Improve cell chemotaxis? Perform an anti-inflammatory/immunomodulatory function? These are all critical questions that need to be answered for each specific tissue that we want to treat with stem cells.

Because of the distinct limitations of current techniques using exogenous cells, the next frontier in cell-based therapy may be methods to stimulate the resident pluripotent cells that are known to exist in many tissues. This "stem cell niche" is felt to be associated with the walls of blood vessels and harbors cells that are likely involved in tissue homeostasis and repair. These cells could potentially be stimulated to induce tissue healing and regeneration in the appropriate circumstances. The research challenge at this time is to identify optimal methods to leverage and stimulate these intrinsic cells.

Another avenue with tremendous potential but that needs further scientific development is the use of induced pluripotent stem cells (iPSC). Creation of these cells is based on the 2006 Nobel Prize concept demonstrating that transfection of adult-derived terminally differentiated cells with four specific genes can "reprogram" the cells to a pluripotent phenotype equivalent to an embryonic stem cell. This approach allows avoidance of the ethical concerns related to the use of embryonic stem cells. A further advantage of the use of iPSCs is that this allows use of the patient's own cells, as the starting cell source can be from a simple peripheral blood sample or a small skin biopsy. However, at this time, further work is required to understand how to eliminate any potential for tumorigenicity of iPSCs. Further challenges include the need to establish methods for large-scale production of GMP-grade cells for clinical use. As manufacturing protocols and facilities are developed for large-scale production of iPSCs, issues related to safety, sterility, and batch-to-batch variability will need to be addressed.

In summary, it is likely that techniques to manipulate and augment the basic biology of various musculoskeletal tissues will represent the next frontier in the treatment of numerous traumatic and degenerative orthopedic conditions. Further basic and translational research will be required to realize the tremendous potential of these approaches.

Am I a Robot or a Surgeon?

32

Iswadi Damasena

When first faced with the question regarding the future of orthopaedic sports medicine, the thought that comes to mind is: Do sports surgeons have a role in this future? Or will science and innovation in sports medicine, which has been progressing at a vast rate, make sports surgeons obsolete?

32.1 Prevention Is Better than Cure!

Research into injury prevention has become a big factor in professional sport. The focus of this research is not only to develop stratergies to prevent injury, but also to enhance recovery and return athletes to the field of play in a shorter period of time. As an example of the commitment to this strategy, in 2017, Manchester United, an English Premier League football club, spent over £30 million on their sports science and development program. But, like any business, they will want to see a return for their investment. And, along with this expenditure comes the ever-higher expectation of improved performance, recovery and rehabilitation. So, with all this investment into sports science and injury reduction, is it likely that athletes will avoid major injury and hence the surgeon's knife altogether? The answer is undoubtedly, no!

In Australia, the last 15 years has seen a 43% rise in ACL surgery. Much of this rise can be attributed to a greater awareness of the injury, improved access to screening and diagnostic imaging, intensive sports specific training programs, a greater number of participants playing sports at an older age, as well as greater access to orthopaedic surgeons. Some of the blame for the rise in injury rates must also be placed on high-level competition, which continues to place greater and greater demands on athletes, which is driven by the appetite of the consumer. A prime example of this is the Australian Football League, which is well known for making

I. Damasena (✉)
Box Hill Hospital, Melbourne, VIC, Australia

© ISAKOS 2020
B. M. Devitt et al. (eds.), *The Future of Orthopaedic Sports Medicine*,
https://doi.org/10.1007/978-3-030-28976-8_32

regular, even annual changes to its rules in order to keep the game fast paced, exciting and in demand. Our athletes are being pushed harder, but has this equated to a greater number of injuries? Of this, I am not sure, but the question must be asked and, indeed, answered. Perhaps importantly, we must ask ourselves the question, as sports surgeons, are we complicit in putting our patients in harm's way?

Sports science has come a long way, and our understanding of what athletes are capable of and how we can improve athletic performance continues to grow. But, if the focus of sports science is purely on the pursuit of better performance does it come at the expense of the best interests or welfare of the athlete? What is the price of the Olympic motto, 'Faster, Higher, Stronger'? Are we pushing our athletes to breaking point to achieve this only to discard them when they inevitably become slower, lower and weaker?

It was only recently that I came across terms such as preventative genomics and nutrigenomics, the art of analysing an athlete's DNA and genetic nutrition profile. These allow sports scientists to study an individual athlete to the point where they can determine an athlete's injury risk profile, perhaps even quantify it, then modify their training, match days and recovery accordingly. My question is, will this extend to the orthopaedic sports surgeon? We are already seeing sporting clubs with high-level athletes request a specific procedure, technique or graft type for their athlete. Should it not be the orthopaedic surgeon who after careful consultation and assessment of the athlete, or more accurately their patient, determines the best treatment for that patient? After all, our years of training teach us to always look after the patient's best interest, not only for their career but also for the rest of their lives. We must be advocates for the patient beyond just getting them back on the field.

Now, I am not suggesting sports science is attempting to alter this philosophy, but if one focuses exclusively on the objective measurement of human performance, the subject, being the person, can be ignored. This is what worries me. As surgeons, our role should not be simply that of a robot fixing a broken part, we need to be doctors and advocates first and foremost.

Who Will Guard the Guardians?

33

Willem M. van der Merwe

Evidence-based medicine (EBM) has been one of the major contributions of increased quality of health care in general and also for our sporting population. EBM is an approach to medical practice intended to optimize decision-making by emphasizing the use of evidence from well-designed and well-conducted research.

This is going to be complicated by an information explosion that can be accumulated so easy with technological availability. Patient-reported outcome measures are becoming more popular for good reason because, at the end of the day, it is how the patient feels that is important and not the treating surgeon's opinion of the job that he has done. Soon every patient will be able to give feedback on the treatment they received and report the outcome on some free application or database. So, we are going to be swamped by information on outcome and how we use this information will drive the treatment options of the future.

Artificial intelligence will dominate the field of medicine in the future because all data can be gathered and analyzed and treatment algorithms can be changed accordingly. This sounds all very plausible, but analyzing these data is only as good as the quality of the data. The question is: Who is gathering these data and who can benefit from it? To manage a database is very expensive, so they will be sponsored by the funders either private or the state. They may want to use these databases to prove that interventional expensive procedures are not warranted or by the manufacturers of the devices may want to prove that these implants warrant the costs.

How we gather all the information and how we analyze it is the biggest challenge we will face in the future, when to ignore "fake news," and when to embrace sound evidence.

Is it time for expert opinion to again play a bigger role. The quality of the data and the way that it is analyzed should be checked and controlled by experts.

W. M. van der Merwe (✉)
University of Cape Town, Cape Town, WC, South Africa

© ISAKOS 2020

B. M. Devitt et al. (eds.), *The Future of Orthopaedic Sports Medicine*,
https://doi.org/10.1007/978-3-030-28976-8_33

Peer-reviewed articles in quality journals have served us well over time and this should count, not open-access journals with poor-quality articles and badly designed methodology.

So, the argument is that fake information just by the sheer volume will drown out the sound evidence, and we will be at the mercy of whoever controls this mountain of information and to their individual motives. We see this in so many other fields, especially politics where rumors and fake news do influence people because human beings want to believe in certain things and will embrace the information that proves it. Populisms is as alive in orthopedics as it is in politics and we all want to believe that some special supplement or procedure will give us our lives back, what is the harm in trying it, as there seems to be so much evidence out there that it works.

You would think that in this dooms-day scenario, the only solution is to bring back the experts to make sense of it all, but I would argue the opposite (surprise), more harm was done when "experts" decided what was good and what was bad, and this information is going to be generated if we like it or not. So, we should embrace it.

The future is artificial intelligence, which will independently analyze all data and information and use algorithms to recommend appropriate treatment. There will be many mistakes and problems, but to use these mistakes to return to expert control medicine will be far more dangerous. Will artificial intelligence and algorithms improve sports orthopedic medicine? I will argue, yes, it has to. And, hopefully 1 day, it will also run our political systems better. Only artificial intelligence can truly be nonbiased, so prepare for it now.

Don't Wait to Worry!

34

James R. Andrews

The field of orthopaedic sports medicine has grown significantly over the past number of decades and continues to expand at an exponential rate. In this particular field, there is a lot of sensationalism by doctors, physical therapists, athletic trainers, coaches, the media and players alike to jump to conclusions before significant evidence is concluded.

The areas of concern in the future of sports medicine are as follows:

- Loss of the art of physical diagnosis.
- Unchecked development of orthobiologics ahead of scientific evidence.
- Robotic surgery and lack of technical training as a true surgeon.
- Demand on the sports surgeon to manage their ever-increasing administrative duties and electronics.
- Decreasing reimbursement and emphasis on economics for our future young surgeons.

The worry over loss of physical exam is not a new problem. It was eloquently presented by Alan G. Apley in an article as far back as 1964 when he said, 'Generations of doctors have warned that the act of clinical examination is in danger of atrophy—and they have always been right. It is a "disuse atrophy" that is particularly common in orthopaedics' [1]. Never is this more true than today, and it is also likely to continue into the future. As radiographs are now also forgotten, the almighty MRI has taken over and diminished the art of the history and physical exam.

I have already seen a decline in orthopaedic residency training, which has put our young surgeons who are entering sports medicine fellowships at a disadvantage in the operating room with respect to technical skill. This has probably occurred due to a shortened working week and the ever-increasing breath of knowledge, which is

J. R. Andrews (✉)
Andrews Institute for Orthopaedics and Sports Medicine, Gulf Breeze, FL, USA

expected of our trainees in sports medicine. In the future, basic training may have to be abbreviated and speciality training lengthened.

The increasing emphasis on performance-based measurements and administrative requirement will take time away from patient care. This will negatively alter the way medicine is practiced and how patients are treated.

The last worry is related to the problems of inevitable and progressively decreasing reimbursement and economic woes!

Our sports medicine surgeons will be challenged to pay more attention to economics becasue of decreasing reimbursement, thus putting what is the best care of our patients at risk. If the desire to increase economics becomes a major force in one's practice, then surely patient care will suffer. Our young physicians should never let economics interfere with doing what is best for their patients!

Overall, the future for our young sports medicine specialist is still bright and unbelievable. They should be proactive and look for answers with a unified voice for future problems. The old adage about 'wait to worry', also known as, 'WTW', is something that should be avoided, and don't be overwhelmed by future problems.

Reference

1. Apley AG. Intelligent Kneemanship. Postgrad Med J. 1964;40:519–20.

Peter MacDonald

Anterior cruciate ligament (ACL) reconstruction is currently the preferred surgery for the treatment of ACL rupture, although this has not always been the case. And, it is possible that trends will move away from this approach in the future. In 2015, van der List et al. described a "shifting phenomena" in ACL tear management, which, in my opinion, is a potential change for younger generations of knee orthopedic surgeons beginning their practices [1].

Decades ago, it was thought that ACL tear could be addressed with a repair of the ligament [2, 3]. The first descriptions of repair date back to 1895 when Robson performed repair surgery on a 41-year-old male [4]. Decades later, numerous authors argued that this kind of treatment was possibly inferior to the increasingly popular ACL reconstruction. High rates of re-tears, persistent instability rates of over 50%, pain, stiffness, and OA were reported for ACL repair based on high-level randomized clinical trials. Because of this, ACL reconstruction became the method of choice for ACL tears in athletes [5–7].

But might we be too dogmatic about the superiority of reconstruction over the repair? Is it possible that we have "shifted" with too much ease from one dogma to another? Are modern techniques and rehabilitation protocols going to evolve along with growth factors and thus increase the attractiveness of repair over reconstruction?

It is important to recognize that not every ACL tear is the same. As van der List et al. described, early studies did not stratify study groups regarding tear location [1]. In fact, even in the 1980s, the authors reported that patients with a proximal tear (stripping from the femoral condyle) may achieve satisfactory results as opposed to other types of tears in which repair is ineffectual [8]. That being said, more authors started to review the literature and challenge the dogma of the 1990s that ACL reconstruction is the only technique that patients should be offered. More recently, evidence based on newer diagnostic techniques like MRI has allowed for the

P. MacDonald (✉)
University of Manitboa, PanAm Clinic, Winnipeg, Manitoba, Canada
e-mail: pmacdonald@panamclinic.com

© ISAKOS 2020
B. M. Devitt et al. (eds.), *The Future of Orthopaedic Sports Medicine*,
https://doi.org/10.1007/978-3-030-28976-8_35

determination of tear pattern. This, coupled with the evolution of arthroscopic techniques, provides the opportunity to not only repair the ACL but also augment it, guarding the repair and allowing faster healing time over conventional reconstruction [9]. These findings, opposite to ACL reconstruction dogma, support that ACL tear treatment should "can" be customized regarding tear pattern as well as the timing of the surgery.

In my opinion, ACL repair should be performed whenever favorable circumstances exist. An acute, proximal tear in a young patient leans me toward ACL repair rather than reconstruction if the athlete is in a situation where recovery time is a huge issue. This is exemplified in two Olympic skiers who recently had ACL repair instead of reconstruction and were able to compete in a 4–5-month time period at the recent games in PyeongChang. Having said that, ACL reconstruction still remains the gold standard for ACL injuries in 2019.

The story of ACL tear management is one of many stories of how paradigms shift in orthopedic surgery. It is also a great example for young orthopedic surgeons of how they can be biased by one paper, which may not necessarily even utilize the best methodology. More than 6000 research articles have been published on ACL in the past 5 years, and as we live in an environment of fake news, my concern is whether our trainees are able to distinguish between sound data and those that are over-represented or generated through poor research quality. And how they let this information influence their decision-making. The above-mentioned examples show us that we, as slightly older and more experienced surgeons, have shifted from one method to another. Hopefully, these kinds of stories will forewarn future physicians.

References

1. van der List JP, DiFelice GS. Primary repair of the anterior cruciate ligament: a paradigm shift. Surgeon. 2017;15(3):161–8.
2. O'Donoghue DH. An analysis of end results of surgical treatment of major injuries to the ligaments of the knee. J Bone Joint Surg Am. 1955;37-A(1):1–13. passim
3. Palmer I. On the injuries to the ligaments of the knee joint: a clinical study. 1938. Clin Orthop Relat Res. 2007;454:17–22. discussion 14
4. Robson AW. VI. Ruptured crucial ligaments and their repair by operation. Ann Surg. 1903;37(5):716–8.
5. Andersson C, Odensten M, Good L, Gillquist J. Surgical or non-surgical treatment of acute rupture of the anterior cruciate ligament. A randomized study with long-term follow-up. J Bone Joint Surg Am. 1989;71(7):965–74.
6. Engebretsen L, Benum P, Fasting O, Molster A, Strand T. A prospective, randomized study of three surgical techniques for treatment of acute ruptures of the anterior cruciate ligament. Am J Sports Med. 1990;18(6):585–90.
7. Feagin JA Jr, Curl WW. Isolated tear of the anterior cruciate ligament: 5-year follow-up study. Am J Sports Med. 1976;4(3):95–100.
8. Strand T, Engesaeter LB, Molster AO, et al. Knee function following suture of fresh tear of the anterior cruciate ligament. Acta Orthop Scand. 1984;55(2):181–4.
9. Taylor SA, Khair MM, Roberts TR, DiFelice GS. Primary repair of the anterior cruciate ligament: a systematic review. Arthroscopy. 2015;31(11):2233–47.

The Big Bang and Its Fall Out

36

Mervyn J. Cross

Being around on the dawn of the 'Big Bang' of Orthopaedic Sports Medicine in 1970, I have witnessed great milestones and advances. I have also witnessed many preventable failures. My biggest worry is that there is a tendency to follow fads, such as the gross failures of intra-articular artificial ligaments, lateral release as the cure of patella instability and the excision of supra-patellar plicae.

International communication now allows us to see and hear what is happening around the world, and this is further supported by an increasing number of journals dedicated to orthopaedic sports medicine. The tendency to publish for publishing's sake, however, is another great concern. The interpretation of data, how they are collected, deciphered and, eventually, presented is a significant worry, as there is still discussion regarding what truly defines 'Evidence-based Medicine'?

My major problem is that we have still not been able to determine the correct graft for anterior cruciate ligament (ACL) reconstruction. We hear very little about the residual problems related to using hamstring tendons for ACL autograft, the loss of muscle amplitude, the scarring and tethering as the tendon regenerates. I still see a great deal of non-anatomical tunnels, particularly with trans-tibial femoral drilling. Indeed, I have come across many examples of nonanatomical tunnels in manuscripts and presentations where good results are expressed. Also, the argument for the conservative treatment of ACL rupture has resurfaced and needs to be explored. In cases of proximal tears, particularly in less active patients, surely there is still a role for bracing alone.

I predict that the operation of '*medial patella ligament*' reconstruction will disappear when we realise that this is simply thickening of the medial structures, which attaches to the patella through a fan-shaped expansion into vastus medialis obliquus muscle. There needs to be more effort to understand that the patella is a sesamoid

M. J. Cross (✉)
Sydney, NSW, Australia
e-mail: mervcros@ozemail.com

© ISAKOS 2020

91

B. M. Devitt et al. (eds.), *The Future of Orthopaedic Sports Medicine*,
https://doi.org/10.1007/978-3-030-28976-8_36

joint and does not have the same structure as that of fixed joints. It is dynamic with seven degrees of freedom and therefore cannot be 'fixed' by tethering a hamstring at two questionable sites on the epicondyle and the patella.

Long-term follow-up is extremely difficult in orthopaedic sports medicine. The population is typically young and mobile and, as such, not easily traceable. Methods to improve the follow-up by giving patients incentives is probably not the best sampling method and is likely to distort the true evidence. But, do we require the most rigorous scientific methods to determine the effectiveness of our treatment? The justification for the majority of orthopaedic sports surgery treatment is generally accepted and easily verified. But, every patient needs to be treated on the merits of each individual case. Consider the example of the treatment of a bucket–handle meniscal tear; this condition can be very effectively managed with the removal of the torn meniscus, but still there are those who have indications for repair. This exemplifies our dilemma, is there ever such an occasion where we can carry out 'a double-blind trial' to determine the best evidence to treat this condition?

A neat algorithm for the treatment of all cases does not exist. Furthermore, the great frustration is that no two humans are alike, and there are even discrepancies in twins. So, what works in one individual may not work in another. The hope for the future is being honest in our research. It is imperative that we dedicated time at our meetings to informed discussion not just didactic talks. We need to embrace social media for our communication, publish our techniques on platforms such as Vumedi but, best of all, make an effort to visit the author in their working environment.

First the Process, Then the Art of Medicine? The Gruyère Theory

37

Philippe Neyret

I would like to start with a small anecdote to underline the value of the process. During a visit to the American Academy of Orthopedic Surgeons meeting in Washington, myself and my wife brought our 10-year-old son to the hospital due to a terrible pain he was suffering in his left heel. The pain had commenced on the plane journey from France to the USA. And, such was his discomfort that he was unable to sleep the night after our arrival despite medication. In the first 6 hours in the hospital, he was attended by four doctors. He had had an MRI, but it had not provided a definitive diagnosis of a tumour, infection or stress fracture, so a biopsy was planned. We were admitted in preparation for the procedure. As part of the admission process, we were asked all of the same questions again, for a fifth time: name, medical history—every piece of information that had already been recorded on file—date of birth, height, weight… Suddenly, a deep discussion between several doctors ensued. The prescribed doses of medication were totally wrong. The dose of the medication did not correlate with the weight of our son. According to the medical staff, this was a near-miss event, but a severe mistake had thankfully been avoided.

This is one example of the benefits of the process and provides an introduction to the Gruyère theory (in fact, it is really the Emmental theory because, as you know, there are no holes in the Gruyère). This concept is used in many industrial procedures in addition to the airline industry. This theory is simple; the more layers of cheese with holes in them that are superimposed on each other, the less chance there is for the holes to align. The simplicity lies in repeating elementary steps as part of a checklist, which are confirmed by a number of individuals at different junctures, the less risk there is of introducing error. This has been widely adopted in the airline industry, and there has been a marked reduction in accidents occurring. But, there is also a contrary view that worries me.

P. Neyret (✉)
Infirmerie Protestante and Centre Albert Trillat, Lyon University, Lyon, France

© ISAKOS 2020 93
B. M. Devitt et al. (eds.), *The Future of Orthopaedic Sports Medicine*,
https://doi.org/10.1007/978-3-030-28976-8_37

Every day we witness doctors tapping on the keyboards of their computers facing the screen during the patient consultation filling in an endless list of boxes. This is even more true of nursing duties where a considerable portion of the time is now spent answering seemingly stupid questions ad infinitum; for example, like the stage of cleaning of the room. While all of the duties are bound to the process, the patient is no longer the centre of concern. Furthermore, from a medico-legal standpoint, it is crucial that all the stages of this process are respected, even more important than the medical art itself. A trend is now emerging whereby there is a harmonisation of surgical practices such that all surgeons adopt the same techniques, according to the same education and are expected to adhere to strict guidelines. To summarise, surgeons will be expected to work in a rigid manner following a standardised management plan with no place of imagination or original thought on how to treat the patient's condition. Surgeons with imagination, creativity, initiative or innovation need not apply. What awaits is an efficient but boring system.

The process is more important than the surgeon and probably more important than the art of medicine. In France, the precautionary principle has been registered in our constitution. The purpose of this is to provide protection for patients from uninformed and arbitrary choices, which are dependent on the whim a surgeon alone. Nevertheless, France has a great history of orthopaedic innovation. If, in the past, some surgeons made disappointing choices, which we were certainly guilty of, we were able to learn from them and make further advances of the back of these errors, which ultimately benefited other patients. In this period where harmonisation, normalisation and mutualisation are key words, I would like to champion for diversity, excellence and innovation.

I am worried about the institutions that want to apply the same rule to our profession that applies to the aircraft pilots. I continue to think that our patients are our pupils. Our mission and our objective deserve better than the simple implementation of the process and guidelines.

The Complexity of a 'Rope'

38

Christopher C. Kaeding

Are there many things more simple than a rope? I can remember at the beginning of my career when most clinicians viewed the anterior cruciate ligament (ACL) as a static check rein that contributed to the mechanical four-bar cross linkage roll/ glide mechanism of the knee joint. It was purely a mechanical view of the ligament, which was viewed basically as a 'rope' that sometimes broke in the knee. As such, when it tore, much research and effort was put into finding a mechanically strong substitute, with mechanically strong fixation at the mechanically isometric insertion sites in the knee. If the ACL rope in the knee tore, all we had to do was replace the rope. These mechanical goals of replacing the ACL dominated for decades and continue to this day.

Prosthetic ACL 'ropes' were tried and failed. Acknowledgement that this was a living rope that needed to biologically incorporate into the knee began, and some effort has been made to enhance this biological process. We have studied PET scans of ACL grafts, and it appears that it takes up to 2 years for grafts to mature as 'living ropes'. There is also an increasing realization that beyond the mechanical dysfunction caused by an ACL tear, that some biological process occurs with an injury to this rope that likely triggers a degenerative process in the knee. This destructive process appears to proceed despite our replacing the mechanical function of the rope. There is an increasing appreciation of the non-mechanical, biological consequences of tearing/repairing this rope and the long-term impact of this biological process on the health of the knee joint.

As part of the evolution of our understanding of the ACL, it became obvious that an ACL injured knee had muscular weakness that needed to be addressed. This evolved into an appreciation of a neuro-muscular impairment of the affected side, as balance and protective reflexes were noted to be compromised. An appreciation of the ACL as an afferent organ began. This 'rope' was starting to look a bit more

C. C. Kaeding (✉)
The Ohio State University, Columbus, OH, USA
e-mail: Christopher.Kaeding@osumc.edu

© ISAKOS 2020
B. M. Devitt et al. (eds.), *The Future of Orthopaedic Sports Medicine*,
https://doi.org/10.1007/978-3-030-28976-8_38

complicated. It then became clear that an ACL injury resulted in the opposite 'normal' lower extremity also being neuro-muscularly impaired. A recent work at my institution has implied that even after 'successful' return to play after an ACL reconstruction, patients have altered motor control pathways in the central nervous system that can be reversed with transcranial electric stimulation of the brain. Much more work is needed, but it appears an ACL injury/reconstruction may result in long-lasting plastic changes in the brain. How can this 'rope' in the distal extremity affect the brain?

Being focused on restoring the mechanical function of this rope, for decades, we focused on KT-1000 and other mechanical metrics for assessing our results of building new ropes. We declared great success in our new ropes stabilizing knees but then found that despite our mechanical success, only about 50% of our 'successes' returned to pre-injury sport activity levels. This was a bit of a surprise to many of us. Looking deeper into why our successes did not return to high levels of activity, we learned that kinesiophobia or fear of re-injury was a major factor in return to play. So now our rope has psychological sequelae after it's injured. Indeed, there are psychologists who would say that by doing preoperative psychological evaluation of our patients that they can better predict our clinical results than we can with all of our knee knowledge. Simply replacing the torn rope does not guarantee success for our patients.

The lesson I outlined above is how grossly we underestimated the complexity of an ACL injury. How naive we appear in retrospect in thinking that the ACL is a simple static rope with a purely mechanical function and a mechanical consequence if torn. We woefully underestimated its neurologic, biological and psychological impact when injured. The situation was far from as simple as we perceived it. As orthopaedists, we are not alone in our failure to appreciate the complexity of the human body and the power of the poorly understood mind–body interaction. I encourage all of our current, especially our young, investigators and critical innovators to remember this, as they pursue the advancement of orthopaedics and to not make the same gross underestimation of the human condition that my generation did in its treatment of a torn 'rope'.

If You Don't Know Where You Are Going,
Any Road Will Take You There!

39

Harvinder Bedi

The delivery of informed consent is considered an essential part of ethical medical practice. It is the process by which a treating health care provider discloses appropriate information to a competent patient so that the patient may make a voluntary choice to accept or refuse treatment [1]. As part of this process, information is conveyed regarding the rationale for and nature of a proposed procedure, the reasonable alternatives to this intervention and the relative risks, benefits and uncertainties of each treatment option.

In order to achieve this, the natural history of the underlying condition must be known. Without this knowledge, it is impossible to assess whether we are helping or harming patients with any given intervention. This issue is of particular relevance in sports medicine given the increasing tendency for athletes to be treated surgically with the expectation that this will hasten recovery and improve outcomes.

It has been highlighted by a number of recent publications and recommendations questioning the widespread use of procedures such as shoulder and knee arthroscopy to treat common conditions such as subacromial pain and degenerative knee arthritis [2, 3].

In my own subspeciality of foot and ankle surgery, there has been an increase in the rates of fixation of injuries of the syndesmosis and Lisfranc joint complex. This is particularly the case for injuries without significant concurrent fracture. The reasons for this are multiple and complex. One of the primary drivers is the improved imaging of ligamentous injuries and the ability to detect subtle changes through MRI scanning with more powerful magnets and better resolution and functional tests such as weight-bearing CT scans. Other factors include improvements in implants and techniques allowing greater ease of surgical performance and technical outcome; the receipt of credit and affirmation for a good outcome in these milder cases when this may only reflect the natural history of the condition; fear of

H. Bedi (✉)
OrthoSport Victoria, Melbourne, VIC, Australia
e-mail: hbedi@osv.com.au

© ISAKOS 2020

97

B. M. Devitt et al. (eds.), *The Future of Orthopaedic Sports Medicine*,
https://doi.org/10.1007/978-3-030-28976-8_39

criticism in the setting of a poor outcome following conservative treatment that may result in a need for late surgery and a delay in return to sport, and finally, the financial incentives to the surgeon and orthopaedic industry that comes with surgical intervention.

Unfortunately, these drivers towards surgery have not been paralleled with an understanding of the outcomes of these injuries when left untreated. In the past, many such injuries were not detected and were therefore left untreated. A proportion would go on to develop poor outcomes, but we have very limited data to determine in whom this would occur.

A cursory literature search of the 2017 PubMed database using the terms 'ankle/ syndesmosis/injury/treatment' revealed interesting results. Eighty-two articles were discovered. Of these, ten were not relevant to the current discussion, 12 were anatomical studies, four were review articles and 57 discussed a multitude of surgical techniques and methods of intra-operative assessment of instability. Notably, only one investigated the long term outcomes of such injuries [4]. There is an obvious bias in the literature toward assessing surgical outcomes and developing new surgical techniques.

Clearly, greater focus needs to be placed on attaining good-quality natural history data. In this regard, Hovelius [5] in a series of publications spanning many years has given us an excellent insight into the outcomes of non-surgically treated primary anterior dislocation of the shoulder. Through this, the early surgical treatment of the condition has emerged and is established as a viable and justifiable option. Without such studies, we leave ourselves open to criticism from the wider community. Furthermore, we need this information to allow us to justify surgical management to our patients and maintain our ethical and intellectual integrity.

References

1. Appelbaum PS. Assessment of patient's competence to consent to treatment. N Engl J Med. 2007;357:1834–40.
2. Schreurs BW, van der Pas SL. No benefit of arthroscopy in subacromial shoulder pain. Lancet. 2018;391(10118):289–91.
3. Siemieniuk RAC, Harris IA, et al. Arthroscopic surgery for degenerative knee arthritis and meniscal tears: a clinical practice guideline. BMJ. 2017;357:j1982. https://doi.org/10.1136/bmj.j1982.
4. Ray R, Koohnejad N, Clement ND, Keenan GF. Ankle fractures with syndesmotic stabilisation are associated with a high rate of secondary osteoarthritis. Foot Ankle Surg. 2019;25(2):180–5. https://doi.org/10.1016/j.fas.2017.10.005.
5. Hovelius L, Rahme H. Primary anterior dislocation of the shoulder: long-term prognosis at the age of 40 years or younger. Knee Surg Sports Traumatol Arthrosc. 2016;24(2):330–42.

What's the Use in Worrying?

40

Peter J. Millett

> *If there is a solution to the problem, then there is no need to worry. If there is no solution to the problem, then there is no need to worry.*
>
> —Dalai Lama

I complete an arthroscopic rotator cuff surgery—my fourth rotator cuff repair this day—and wonder, "What is next? What will be the next unsolved sports medicine problem to tackle?" During my relatively brief career in orthopaedics, I have seen the evolution of this procedure from an open deltoid-splitting repair with prolonged and oftentimes capricious outcomes to a reproducible, minimally invasive arthroscopic procedure, with reliable fixation techniques and predictable outcomes. In most instances, we can fix rotator cuff tears—all shapes and sizes—through small arthroscopic portals, using biomechanically optimized repair constructs that allow patients to recover faster and back to normal levels of function. That is amazing!

Worry can be defined as: "giving way to anxiety or unease; to allow one's mind to dwell on difficulty or troubles."

For a number of reasons, I don't think it is time to worry. For one, given the rapidity of innovation in our field, in my opinion, there is really no need to worry about the future of orthopaedic sports medicine. Orthopaedic sports medicine is, in my opinion, THE most exciting area of medicine and one that is on sound footing and looks to be so for some time. There is so much to look forward to. With exciting new technologies that allow patients to heal faster and have more predictable outcomes, demographic trends that necessitate keeping people active longer, strong

P. J. Millett (✉)
The Steadman Clinic, Vail, CO, USA
e-mail: drmillett@thesteadmanclinic.com

© ISAKOS 2020

B. M. Devitt et al. (eds.), *The Future of Orthopaedic Sports Medicine*,
https://doi.org/10.1007/978-3-030-28976-8_40

research programs that are now focusing not only on basic science but also on clinical results and patient-reported outcomes, the future of sports medicine has never been brighter.

Our future, however, is dependent on and only as good as the people who create it. There is little to worry about here too. From my observations, I believe we are fortunate to have a highly capable and very inspired, new generation of surgeons entering sports medicine. Orthopaedics is no doubt attracting the best and the brightest. It has been said that "one of the best ways to predict the future is to create it," and I believe the orthopaedic sports medicine community, which has some of the brightest minds and which is, moreover, attracting the brightest minds from medical school and from the research community, will no doubt create our brighter future. From my own personal experience, I remain in awe at the talent pool. For example, we recently completed our Sports Medicine fellowship interviews, and I was truly astonished at and humbled by the breadth and depth of skilled, smart and talented young surgeons who are eagerly entering our field. Each year I ask, "How can so many amazing applicants be applying? Where are they coming from?" They are consistently from the best universities, medical schools and residency training programs, in the top percentile on their licensing exams, and yet they remain genuinely humble, hungry, and passionate about sports medicine. They are the anti-thesis of the stereotypical disengaged millennial generation and instead are energized, engaged, motivated, smart and caring. They will no doubt propel our specialty to places of which we can only dream.

The last 20 years have been an exciting time in sports medicine—the advent of the arthroscope, the growth of sports in society, the demographic shifts in which people stay active longer, innovations in materials sciences, and the emergence of sports medicine as a sub-specialty of orthopaedic surgery. All these factors have impacted the field. We have treatments that were unimaginable to those of the last generation.

But that doesn't mean we can rest on our laurels, for there is much work to be done and many unsolved problems that face us and our patients. Despite these challenges, I believe that orthopaedic sports medicine, which attracts the brightest minds and the most motivated people, will continue to innovate with new technology and better treatments for our patients, and that this creativity should keep us from worrying for some time.

High-Technology Technicians Versus Bedside Doctors

41

Joan C. Monllau

The American Academy of Orthopaedic Surgeons defines orthopaedic surgery as *'the medical specialty that includes the investigation, preservation and restoration of the form and function of the extremities, spine and associated structures by medical, surgical, and physical means.'* Besides trauma of the musculoskeletal system, the current speciality deals with growth disorders and developmental issues around the skeleton, degenerative arthritis and congenital deformities. To that end, the speciality has been undergoing a process of refinement overtime, and orthopaedic surgeons currently use technology extensively and a great number of modern devices in their daily practice.

In recent decades, minimally invasive surgery, arthroscopy, navigation, robotics and, of late, biological treatments have progressively become more and more widespread. These advances have made some orthopaedic procedures easier, more cost-effective and contributed to improving patient satisfaction. These technologies will probably change if not replace most of the activities orthopaedic surgeons engage in to do their work.

The aim of this essay is to review the current trends in practice and the possible evolution of our specialty in the forthcoming years as seen from this author's perspective.

41.1 Reducing or Eliminating the Hospital Stay: The New Paradigm

In many countries in Europe where the public system is strong, many hospitals are running at overcapacity and must cancel elective surgery, like joint replacement operations, amongst others, due to a lack of beds. In that sense, the

J. C. Monllau (✉)
Department of Orthopaedic Surgery, Hospital del Mar, Barcelona, Spain
e-mail: JMonllau@parcdesalutmar.cat

© ISAKOS 2020   101
B. M. Devitt et al. (eds.), *The Future of Orthopaedic Sports Medicine*,
https://doi.org/10.1007/978-3-030-28976-8_41

potential to liberate hospital beds by fast tracking operations facilitated by new technologies is quite significant and appears feasible without compromising patient care. In the last 30 years, arthroscopic surgery has emerged from incipience to full maturity. To this end, arthroscopic procedures, believed to be impossible a few years ago, like reshaping a femoral head, are currently done as day care surgeries.

Apart from saving money, some additional patient benefits of that policy may be in keeping them in a safer and more comfortable environment to decrease the risk of infection by the more virulent hospital bacteria.

41.2   From Navigation to Robotics

Navigation was introduced into orthopaedic surgery in the early 1990s for use in the planning and optimal positioning of joint replacement implants. Due to the evidence in support of navigation surgery over conventional surgery, robotics has been introduced as one next logical step. There is now good evidence that prostate and other forms of abdominal surgery are safer and more effective when robots are used. Both patients and doctors have so far shown great interest and enthusiasm for surgery assisted by robots. However, as to whether orthopaedic implants, like prostheses, that have been precisely positioned by the robot reduce the failure rate has not yet been proven. These doubts and concerns will be solved in forthcoming years. In the meantime, surgeons should balance the potential advantages of this technology with the considerable investment robotic equipment requires.

Last but not least significant, there is the issue of liability. Even robots can make mistakes. In that case, who will be liable? Will it be the surgeon who is supervising the procedure or the robot manufacturer? This significant issue should be addressed and clarified before massively extending their use.

41.3   Biological Treatments: The New Frontier

In the last decade, there has been a massive shift towards the use of biological treatments. These strategies seek to enhance musculoskeletal tissue regeneration and repair by modulating the microenvironment at the injury site. The use of platelet-rich plasma (PRP), stem cell therapy and scaffolds has considerable therapeutic potential, but their current role is somewhat controversial, particularly in the case of PRP. The development of cell-based therapies seeded, or not, on the appropriate scaffolds currently appears to be a much more refined and reliable approach.

The most suitable cells and scaffolds with the addition of selected growth factors will be defined in the next 20 years. It is likely that this approach will be common to most musculoskeletal injuries including those of cartilage, meniscus, ligaments, tendons and even bones.

I feel patients would still like human orthopaedic surgeons to be around them during the treatment process, as a large component of the orthopaedic surgeon–patient relationship is based on communication and confidence. Therefore, I do not see robots replacing orthopaedic surgeons in the future.

However, as new technologies may contribute to increasing the accuracy of techniques and the safety of our patients, effort needs to be made to conciliate the apparent paradox of a surgeon technician spending most of the time in the outpatient clinic looking at his/her laptop instead of talking to and examining the patient. This will be a challenge to overcome in the forthcoming decades.

Surgery Is Overvalued and Rehabilitation Undervalued Following Anterior Cruciate Ligament Injury

42

Christian J. Barton

It is possible to return to play with complete non-operative management, within 8 weeks, following a complete ACL injury in professional football—Learning point from a 2015 *British Medical Journal* case report [1]

Rupturing an anterior cruciate ligament (ACL) has undoubted significance to an individual's athletic pursuits and remaining life. Early surgical management is commonly encouraged and supported by health system funding. The recovery period is long and arduous. The two primary surgical approaches are hamstring- and patellar-tendon autografts, but the more effective of the two, along with the potential value of many other surgical approaches, remains unclear.

Surgical reconstruction following ACL injury is likely over-valued in many contexts. Although there is debate, the more prevalent belief among the medical and surgical community is that surgical reconstruction is necessary to facilitate return to sport and reduce the risk of osteoarthritis development [2]. After surgery, athletes are typically told their knee is fixed, and in time, they will return to sport. However, compelling evidence tells us successful return to sport rates are sub-optimal (65%) [3] and re-rupture rates high (23%) [4]. Additionally, surgical reconstruction results in iatrogenic trauma to the knee and subsequent increased risk of injury to donor sites (hamstring or patellar tendon). Strikingly, 98% of athletes undergoing reconstruction expect little-to-no increase in their risk of developing knee osteoarthritis [5]. However, approximately 40% will develop radiographic knee osteoarthritis 14–15 years following an ACL injury [6], and there is no difference in long-term

C. J. Barton (✉)
La Trobe Sport and Exercise Medicine Research Centre, School of Allied Health, La Trobe University, Bundoora, VIC, Australia

Department of Surgery, St Vincent's Hospital, University of Melbourne, Fitzroy, VIC, Australia
e-mail: christian@completesportscare.com.au

© ISAKOS 2020
B. M. Devitt et al. (eds.), *The Future of Orthopaedic Sports Medicine*,
https://doi.org/10.1007/978-3-030-28976-8_42

rates of osteoarthritis between those who receive surgery and those who do not [6]. The so-called "surgical fix" is far from a fix.

The only high-quality randomised controlled trial comparing early surgical reconstruction to rehabilitation with the option of delayed surgery (KANON trial) reported no difference in function, symptoms, radiographic findings and physical activity levels between groups for up to 5 years post-injury in non-elite athletes [7]. Despite this, non-surgical management following ACL injury in many health settings is rare. Engrained culture, along with medical and community beliefs, prevents similar research in elite settings. However, a recent BMJ case report highlights a full return to sport within 8 weeks of a complete ACL rupture in an elite English Premier League player [1]. Importantly, the player was reported to remain problem-free at 18 months follow-up.

42.1   Rehabilitation Is Undervalued

The ability to perform functional tasks requires a strong and resilient musculoskeletal system, not one ligament. Optimising physical performance appears to be the key to achieving outstanding outcomes following ACL injury and preventing the need for delayed reconstruction in those starting with rehabilitation alone [8]. Yet, participation in good-quality rehabilitation and objective return to sport screening is alarmingly low, with 45% of community-level athletes discontinuing supervised rehabilitation by 3 months post-ACLR [9]. Subsequently, restoration of the numerous functional impairments seen in athletes following ACL injury is made extremely challenging. Based on contemporary exercise science knowledge, a short rehabilitation period cannot be adequate. The current undervaluing of graded and progressive rehabilitation by medical professionals, the public and health funding models is likely driving current high rates of failed return to sport and re-rupture. This must change.

How to change culture and engrained beliefs about ACL injury management should be our biggest worry. It is time to stop wasting money and resources researching how to optimise surgical approaches to improve long-term outcomes and return to sport. This waste includes an alarming resurgence in experimenting with synthetic ligaments and more recent experiments with animal (e.g. kangaroo) tendons. We must stop the common blind recommendation that an ACL injury needs to be 'fixed' with a reconstruction and endeavour to understand those who do and do not need surgical reconstruction.

Based on evidence, it makes sense to trial non-surgical management first. Yet, in many health settings, consideration to non-surgical management is rare, and there is a clear lack of acceptance by some that it might be successful. Our language when discussing treatment options also matters enormously. If we continue to call the non-surgical approach 'conservative management,' incentive for athletes and medical professionals to change practice will remain low. The term 'conservative' must be abandoned, or quality exercise rehabilitation cannot compete with surgery in relation to perceived value. Even in the case of early reconstruction, a well-designed graded and progressive rehabilitation program should be facilitated, despite its arduous and intensive process. Considering the rarity of this, the importance of quality rehabilitation requires united promotion from all health professionals and the community.

Rehabilitation is of high value only if we get it right. Patient buy-in through quality patient education, goal-setting and enhancing motivation through feedback and repeated functional testing is vital. Progressive exercise and 'sport-specific rehabilitation' based on accepted resistance training principles and patient needs must be guided to prepare each athlete for a return to sport. These approaches are associated with outstanding outcomes and used successfully by world leaders in ACL rehabilitation [8]. Whether surgical reconstruction is chosen or not, we must stop overvaluing surgery and undervaluing rehabilitation following ACL injury.

References

1. Weiler R, Monte-Colombo M, Mitchell A, Haddad F. Non-operative management of a complete anterior cruciate ligament injury in an English premier league football player with return to play in less than 8 weeks: applying common sense in the absence of evidence. BMJ Case Rep. 2015;2015.
2. Marx RG, Jones EC, Angel M, Wickiewicz TL, Warren RF. Beliefs and attitudes of members of the American Academy of Orthopaedic surgeons regarding the treatment of anterior cruciate ligament injury. Arthroscopy. 2003;19(7):762–70.
3. Ardern CL, Taylor NF, Feller JA, Webster KE. Fifty-five per cent return to competitive sport following anterior cruciate ligament reconstruction surgery: an updated systematic review and meta-analysis including aspects of physical functioning and contextual factors. Br J Sports Med. 2014;48(21):1543–52.
4. Wiggins AJ, Grandhi RK, Schneider DK, Stanfield D, Webster KE, Myer GD. Risk of secondary injury in younger athletes after anterior cruciate ligament reconstruction: a systematic review and meta-analysis. Am J Sports Med. 2016;44(7):1861–76.
5. Feucht MJ, Cotic M, Saier T, et al. Patient expectations of primary and revision anterior cruciate ligament reconstruction. Knee Surg Sports Traumatol Arthrosc. 2016;24(1):201–7.
6. von Porat A, Roos EM, Roos H. High prevalence of osteoarthritis 14 years after an anterior cruciate ligament tear in male soccer players: a study of radiographic and patient relevant outcomes. Ann Rheum Dis. 2004;63(3):269–73.
7. Frobell RB, Roos HP, Roos EM, Roemer FW, Ranstam J, Lohmander LS. Treatment for acute anterior cruciate ligament tear: five year outcome of randomised trial. Br J Sports Med. 2015;49(10):700.
8. Grindem H, Risberg MA, Eitzen I. Two factors that may underpin outstanding outcomes after ACL rehabilitation. Br J Sports Med. 2015;49(22):1425.
9. Ebert JR, Edwards P, Yi L, et al. Strength and functional symmetry is associated with post-operative rehabilitation in patients following anterior cruciate ligament reconstruction. Knee Surg Sports Traumatol Arthrosc. 2018;26(8):2353–61.

The Professional Responsibility of Orthopaedic Sports Medicine Surgeons as Advocates for Sports Injury Prevention

43

Christopher Vertullo

Health advocacy has been defined as *'Action by a physician to promote those social, economic, educational, and political changes that ameliorate the suffering and threats to human health and well-being that he or she identifies through his or her professional work and expertise'* [1]. *Advocacy has also been proposed to form a principle component of being a medical professional and of professionalism itself* [2–4].

The burden of musculoskeletal disease is both significant to society as a whole and on those individuals afflicted. Obesity and lower limb sports injuries are both specifically linked to an increased risk of the development of knee osteoarthritis, particularly in an ageing population. The burden of disease with lower limb injury, particularly anterior cruciate ligament (ACL) tears and meniscal injury, falls most heavily on the young. This is on a background of an increasing incidence of sports injuries and ACL tears [5], with sports injuries in some countries now accounting for a greater proportion of hospital admissions than road traffic trauma [6]. While orthopaedic sports medicine surgeons have achieved great strides in musculoskeletal restoration after sports injury as healers, this focus on biomedical management of the injured young athlete has unfortunately somewhat disregarded the at-risk but so far uninjured youth athlete.

Over the last 20 years, there has been increasing recognition that many lower limb sports injuries are not just inevitable; they are in fact 50–80% preventable via cost-effective inexpensive neuromuscular agility training programs [7–9]. Consequently, orthopaedic sports medicine surgeons have a profound professional responsibility to be prominent health advocates for lower limb sports injury prevention. Large national or international medical societies such as ISAKOS or a coalition of like-minded organizations are much more effective health advocates than a large number of small independent societies or individuals, no matter how

C. Vertullo (✉)
GCORE, Griffith University, Gold Coast, QLD, Australia

Knee Research Australia, Gold Coast, QLD, Australia

© ISAKOS 2020
B. M. Devitt et al. (eds.), *The Future of Orthopaedic Sports Medicine*,
https://doi.org/10.1007/978-3-030-28976-8_43

prominent they are. A national example of this coalition approach is the 'safe sports for kids' initiative led by the Australiana Orthopaedic Association (AOA), which is a large group of clinical and sporting stakeholders advocating for a National Sports Injury Prevention Program [10]. Large medical societies typically have the resources and depth to conduct multiple-year advocacy programs within their areas of specific clinical concern.

An effectively designed and implemented advocacy program is vital to achieve its public health objectives. Firstly, the objectives need to be clearly defined, for example, 'A 50% reduction in acute ACLR injuries in 12- to 25-year-olds playing high-risk team sports by 2022' is a more easily implemented and measurable outcome than, 'to reduce knee osteoarthritis from ACL tears'. Once the objectives of the advocacy are defined, the strategies to fulfil those goals can then be designed. The first strategy to attempt is a 'win-win' outcome, where advocates work with identified key stakeholders, such as government health officials and sporting codes, who can be seen as leading the initiative rather than being forced into them [11]. One example of this is the aforementioned AOA's Safe Sports for Kids initiative.

Opposition and barriers to health advocacy by clinicians can come from government, industry, community interests groups and individuals [11]. Another common barrier is indifference, with some issues being neglected because they are regarded as unimportant or inevitable. One such public health issue that was initially disregarded, and unfortunately still is in some developing nations, is road accident trauma (RTA), which initially faced the barriers of indifference, belief of inevitability and then opposition from government, the vehicle manufacturing industry, motoring interest groups and individual motorists. Today, largely, as a result of health advocacy in many developed nations, RTA rates are declining [12]. An awareness that many sports injuries are preventable is lacking in the community, as many, particularly the media, regard sports injury as just bad luck rather than poor preparation.

Identification of mechanisms to influence key stakeholders is vital [13], as are the recognition of the strengths and weaknesses of your position as well as that of the oppositions. For instance, with sports injury prevention, it is important to remain 'pro-sport' for its overall lifestyle and health benefits, such as avoidance of obesity and mental health, to avoid being labelled as 'nanny-state' paternalism [14]. Framing the issue of reducing sports injury as vital to the future sporting success of the individual, team, region or nation is one method to avoid opposition and involve key sporting stakeholders. Injured champions can't play, and they can't win.

Interaction with the media is best undertaken with recognition of what the media requires in a story. Firstly, it has to be new and compelling from a reputable source to be 'news'. Secondly, the issue is more likely to gain traction if it is personalisable to the listener. Journalists much prefer stories about real injured young athletes undergoing surgery, preferably with photos or vision, to epidemiologists dryly reporting increases in hospitalisation per 100,000 sports participants. It is for this reason the surgeon who talks about 'their' patients is more a powerful health advocate in the media than a non-clinician; however, scientific evidence to back up the truth of the message is always required. Involvement of media experts and media-training of the surgeon-spokesperson or 'talent' is vital to enable media-repeatable sound bites framing the program's objectives [15] as part of a well-planned strategy [11].

In conclusion, coherent international advocacy of sports injury prevention is lacking despite the increasing burden of preventable knee osteoarthritis. Large international medical societies such as ISAKOS have an important professional responsibility to be more than just a society of healers of the injured but also advocates for effective well-considered prevention programs amongst the at-risk but so far uninjured young athlete.

References

1. Earnest MA, Wong SL, Federico SG. Perspective: physician advocacy: what is it and how do we do it? Acad Med. 2010;85(1):63–7.
2. Luft LM. The essential role of physician as advocate: how and why we pass it on. Can Med Educ J. 2017;8(3):e109–16.
3. Riddick FA. The code of medical ethics of the American Medical Association. Ochsner J. 2003;5(2):6–10.
4. Royal Australasian College of Surgeons: Advocacy [Internet]. 2016. https://www.surgeons.org/for-the-public/racs-global-health/advocacy/#. Accessed 29 July 2018.
5. Zbrojkiewicz D, Vertullo C, Grayson JE. Increasing rates of anterior cruciate ligament reconstruction in young Australians, 2000-2015. Med J Aust. 2018;208(8):354–8.
6. Finch CF, Kemp JL, Clapperton AJ. The incidence and burden of hospital-treated sports-related injury in people aged 15+ years in Victoria, Australia, 2004–2010: a future epidemic of osteoarthritis? Osteoarthritis Cartilage [Internet]. 2015. http://linkinghub.elsevier.com/retrieve/pii/S1063458415002095. Accessed 3 May 2015.
7. Caraffa A, Cerulli G, Projetti M, Aisa G, Rizzo A. Prevention of anterior cruciate ligament injuries in soccer. Knee Surg Sports Traumatol Arthrosc. 1996;4(1):19–21.
8. Sadoghi P, von Keudell A, Vavken P. Effectiveness of anterior cruciate ligament injury prevention training programs. J Bone Joint Surg Am. 2012;94(9):769–76. https://doi.org/10.2106/JBJS.K.00467.
9. Lewis DA, Kirkbride B, Vertullo CJ, Gordon L, Comans TA. Comparison of four alternative national universal anterior cruciate ligament injury prevention programme implementation strategies to reduce secondary future medical costs. Br J Sports Med. 2016;52(4):277–82.
10. Safe Sports for Kids: A National Youth Sports Injury Prevention Initiative [Internet]. Safe Sport for Kids. 2015. http://www.safesport.org.au/. Accessed 29 July 2018.
11. Chapman S. Advocacy for public health: a primer. J Epidemiol Community Health. 2004;58(5):361–5.
12. Ernstberger A, Joeris A, Daigl M, Kiss M, Angerpointner K, Nerlich M, et al. Decrease of morbidity in road traffic accidents in a high income country – an analysis of 24,405 accidents in a 21 year period. Injury. 2015;46:S135–43.
13. Sethi MK, Obremskey A, Sathiyakumar V, Gill JT, Mather RC. The evolution of advocacy and orthopaedic surgery. Clin Orthop Relat Res. 2013;471(6):1873–8.
14. Ten Worst Nanny Sate Policies [Internet]. 2016. https://ipa.org.au/publications-ipa/ipa-review-articles/10-worst-nanny-state-policies. Accessed 29 July 2018.
15. The Project - Channel Ten, Australia. "Kids Knees are Collapsing" [Internet]. 2018. https://www.facebook.com/TheProjectTV/videos/kids-knees-collapsing/10155485648118441/. Accessed 29 July 2018.

Digitalization and Machine Learning

44

Kristoffer W. Barfod

The largest threat to orthopaedic sports medicine might also be the greatest opportunity, namely the integration of artificial intelligence in our profession by digitalization and machine learning. Digitalization is incorporation of digital technology into all aspects of everyday life of the patient and the physician. Machine learning is a way for artificial intelligence to progressively improve performance on specific tasks based on the big data collected in the digitalized world.

Machine algorithms will be able to recognize abnormalities in three-dimensional MRI scans and three-dimensional motion analysis patterns, and from this, suggest surgical corrections. With time, robot (assisted) surgery will take over the most essential parts of the operations and reduce the surgeon to a highly qualified operator. It has already started with joint replacement and reconstruction procedures where robot-assisted surgery has been tested with varying success. Don't be fooled by the early teething problems with this new technology. With gradual refinements and improvement, robotic surgery will grow into the future of sports surgery. Difficult reconstructions like knee and patella alignment in the young dysplastic knee will be revolutionized. The machine algorithms will be able to include data on pelvic tilt, femoral anteversion, leg axis, tibial torsion, trochlear dysplasia and patella shape. On top of this, muscular strength and direction of force transmission can be incorporated into the models. With time, robot (assisted) trochleoplasty, based on a full extremity scan and gait analysis, will allow for reconstruction procedures optimizing joint congruency, limb axis and rotational alignment.

On a public health level, digitalization and technology have contributed significantly to inactivity of our population, which has, in turn, developed into a major health issue. Physical inactivity is considered the most important major threat to public health by the World Health Organization, as physical inactivity is known to

K. W. Barfod (✉)
Department of Orthopedic Surgery, Sports Orthopedic Research Center—Copenhagen,
Copenhagen University Hospital Hvidovre, Copenhagen, Denmark
e-mail: kbarfod@dadlnet.dk

© ISAKOS 2020
B. M. Devitt et al. (eds.), *The Future of Orthopaedic Sports Medicine*,
https://doi.org/10.1007/978-3-030-28976-8_44

lead to obesity, metabolic syndrome and diabetes. The Orthopaedic Sports Medicine physician will need to expand his/her skills to play a clear role in counselling and treatment of this public health threat.

Injuries among young obese patients will increase, making it difficult for them to exercise and lose weight. It is a vicious circle that needs new treatment strategies to allow for better health and increased life expectancy. We need to define treatment algorithms and cooperate in interdisciplinary teams to help this patient group.

We can also expect an increasing proportion of young obese patients with arthritis seeking help to relieve their pain and allow for an increased physical activity level. The young age at onset of arthritis puts extra demand on implant survival in high-demand patients.

At the same time, machine learning will take over a larger part of diagnostics and counselling of patients. It will enable patients to diagnose their own diseases and make them better informed when consulting the surgeon. It might develop into a threat to the sports medicine physician that will lose patients to the digitalized physician. However, it will more likely develop into a working tool for the sports medicine physician, as the patient will rely on the 'human factor' when seeking advice concerning their health.

All in all, the future for orthopaedic sports medicine is challenging and exciting. With an ever-ageing and increasingly overweight population, we will have plenty to do.

David Pitts

What is orthopaedic sports medicine? Where do its practitioners fit into the emerging community of sports and exercise medicine (SEM), and most importantly, what role should the speciality play on the international stage?

If you pose the first of these questions to some (many?) surgically focused SEM professionals, you will probably get the sort of answers that reflect the "Wikipedia" approach.

> "sports medicine" … encompasses a group of professionals from various disciplines whose focus is the health of an athlete…. Orthopaedic sports medicine is the investigation, preservation, and restoration by medical, surgical, and rehabilitative means to all structures of the musculoskeletal system affected by athletic activity [1].

Is it all about the treatment of injured athletes? As the conversation progresses, the picture emerges of doctors who see themselves rushing on to the field of play to rescue David Beckham's Achilles tendon, Wayne Rooney's fractured metatarsal or some similarly high-profile sportsperson with an injury that disrupts a televised competitive event. So, it's not just athletes but 'elite' athletes?

Why should anyone be worried about this?

Firstly, because this caricature undersells the clinical realities. When you ask the same people about their day-to-day practice, they readily admit that they are more likely to see the soccer-mom who twisted her ankle sprinting along a muddy touchline than the elite athlete injured in actual combat. And for the most part orthopaedic sports medicine is just one of the things they do in their daily job as an orthopaedic surgeon.

Secondly, just because many patients seeking help are not athletes doesn't mean that sports orthopaedics has nothing to contribute to their treatment. Wayne Rooney chose the removable plastic cast over the traditional plaster cast. 'Removable plastic

D. Pitts (✉)
Cupar, UK
e-mail: dpitts@creativelearning.co.uk

© ISAKOS 2020

115

B. M. Devitt et al. (eds.), *The Future of Orthopaedic Sports Medicine*,
https://doi.org/10.1007/978-3-030-28976-8_45

casts provide compression which limits swelling and the rocker sole allows early weight bearing … Research has shown that early weight bearing helps to speed fracture healing…' [2] No doubt, in the weeks that followed Rooney's 2006 injury, every patient attending Manchester's fracture clinics asked why they couldn't have a cast like the one Wayne Rooney had.

Thirdly, because orthopaedic sports medicine risks missing strategic opportunities to influence patient care on a widespread basis if it fails to see the bigger picture.

According to the International Federation of Sports Medicine [3], Sports Medicine is a discipline… '…embodying theoretical and practical medicine which examines the influence of exercise, training and sports, as well as the lack of exercise, on healthy and unhealthy people of all ages to produce results that are conducive to prevention, therapy and rehabilitation as well as beneficial for the athlete himself'.

The number of athletes (elite or otherwise) is dwarfed by the vast numbers of sufferers from osteoporosis, arthritis, type 2 diabetes, war injuries. All of these patients may benefit in some way from the knowledge and skills of SEM doctors in general or orthopaedic sports surgeons in particular. For that benefit to be a reality, three key elements need to be highlighted in the orthopaedic sports paradigm:

45.1 Perspective

Athletes (especially elite athletes) are a (young, fit, healthy…) means to developing treatments for wider populations of patients, not the sole end of treatment in themselves. This is absolutely not to deny their needs as patients, but their celebrity should illuminate rather than obscure wider needs. Athletes can be partners, not just patients.

45.2 Prevention

Diagnosis of an injury or condition and its treatment plan should contribute wherever possible to the prevention of such injuries in the future. In a 2016 Orthopaedic Sports Medicine conference [4], only three of the 21 papers presented (35 min of 12.5 h of conference time) focused on prevention.

45.3 Advocacy

At the heart of a medical vocation is the doctor's role as advocate for the patient. Orthopaedic sports practitioners have a key role to play as patient advocates in both innovation and education. The 'technology and tools' focus in orthopaedics is arguably responsible for much of its success as a speciality. This goes beyond the plates, screws, implants and the tools to manipulate them to the complexities and depth of the network of international educational programmes that draws the community together. It is one thing to build the scientific platform that identifies the need for the plastic removable cast that returned Wayne Rooney so efficiently to the soccer pitch. It is quite another leap of advocacy to campaign for that cast to be produced in sufficient numbers and at sufficiently low cost that landmine victims in Afghanistan can benefit from it in the same way.

A 2019 Orthopaedics Sports education conference describes its focus as 'Keeping Patients Active Through Biologics, Rehabilitation& Contemporary Surgical Techniques' [5].

This vision that highlights the focus on patients may be one that enables orthopaedic sports medicine to re-affirm its holistic mission to care for all patients, not just the athletes?

References

1. Orthopaedic Sports Medicine in Wikipedia. https://en.wikipedia.org/wiki/Orthopaedic_sports_medicine. Accessed 31 Aug 2018.
2. https://www.physioroom.com/sports/injury_case_studies/metatarsal_fracture_rooney.php. Accessed 31 Aug 2018.
3. McCrory P. What is sports and exercise medicine? Br J Sports Med. 2006;40(12):955–7.
4. American Orthopaedic Society for Sports Medicine, Saturday, March 5, 2016. https://www.aaos.org/uploadedFiles/PreProduction/anmeet/AOSSM.pdf. Accessed 31 Aug 2018.
5. American Orthopaedic Society for Sports Medicine, sub title of 2019 Education conference. https://www.aaos.org/1903243/. Accessed 31 Aug 2018.

Why Are ACL Injury Prevention Programs Not Being Implemented More Widely?

46

Robert G. Marx

Anterior cruciate ligament (ACL) injuries are extremely common and lead to devastating consequences including recovery time and time away from sport, risks of surgery for patients who elect to undergo ACL reconstruction, and increased risk of osteoarthritis of the knee. There is now significant evidence demonstrating that the risk of this injury can be dramatically decreased by doing an exercise program emphasizing core strength, balance, proprioception, and safe movement patterns. Despite the medical evidence that has accumulated, these programs are generally not widely used in most places in the world.

The reason for this is likely multifactorial. In general, people do not like taking action that requires discipline and effort in order to prevent medical problems. For example, patients generally prefer to take medication to reduce their cholesterol, rather than severely modifying their diet to achieve a similar result.

ACL injury prevention programs are different. The decision to implement is made by the coaches and training staff, rather than the athletes. Nevertheless, the team leaders often have other priorities and may have difficulty relating the exercises to injuries prevented and keeping their athletes on the field.

The best approach to disseminating this information in order to have athletes best prepared for injury-free practice and competition remains unknown. This is a critical issue that will be faced by sports medicine physicians and public health advocates in the future.

A similar example is seatbelts that improve safety, when traveling in a vehicle. A few decades ago, seatbelts didn't exist, and only more recently have they become very commonly used. With the passage of time, injury prevention strategies can become routine and standard. We must improve sports injury prevention strategies to arrive at a similar level of compliance. As surgeons, we can repair ACL-injured knees one at a time; however, with wide implementation of injury prevention strategies, we can save thousands of knees without lifting a knife.

R. G. Marx (✉)
Hospital for Special Surgery, Weill Cornell Medical College, New York, NY, USA
e-mail: MarxR@HSS.EDU

© ISAKOS 2020

119

B. M. Devitt et al. (eds.), *The Future of Orthopaedic Sports Medicine*,
https://doi.org/10.1007/978-3-030-28976-8_46

Think of the Children

47

Timothy Lording

The issue that worries me most in orthopaedic sports medicine is the fate of the adolescent athlete with an ACL injury.

I will never forget the very first patient I saw in private practice when I returned from fellowship 4 years ago: a 14-year-old boy who was a promising Australian Rules footballer who had represented his state team for his age group. He tore his ACL in a non-contact incident. He had a family history of ACL rupture, with his father having torn both during his playing days. When I explained the statistics for re-injury after reconstruction, and for contralateral knee injury at his age, his father fainted, literally out cold on the floor of the consulting room.

And the truth be told, the statistics are pretty horrifying. Local research from Melbourne has shown a 29% chance of re-rupture of the ACL graft or contralateral ACL injury in patients under 20 years of age [1]. A positive family history (let alone a family history of bilateral injury) doubled the odds of further injury. And these are the outcomes in the most experienced and respected hands in town, not some young surgeon just home from fellowship.

Australia has the highest rate of ACL reconstruction in the world [2]. The peak incidence for females is from 15 to 19 years of age, while the fastest annual growth in incidence is in those aged under 14 years. Whilst reconstruction rates are highest in males, females who participate in high-risk sports are reportedly at higher risk of ACL injury [3], and I suspect that the recent popularization of women's Australian Rules football (footy) we are currently seeing in Melbourne will lead to a significant and demonstrable increase in the injury burden amongst young girls. Indeed, I have recently reconstructed the ACLs of two sisters, aged 15 and 17 years, just 6 weeks apart after their footy injuries. They were referred to me by their coach, who I reconstructed last year after her footy injury.

These girls have a 13-year-old brother and an 11-year-old sister who both play footy too, and I consider them at extreme risk for ACL injury. Ideally, I would like

T. Lording (✉)
Melbourne Orthopaedic Group, Melbourne, Australia

© ISAKOS 2020
B. M. Devitt et al. (eds.), *The Future of Orthopaedic Sports Medicine*,
https://doi.org/10.1007/978-3-030-28976-8_47

to send the whole family to an ACL prevention program, but where to send them? There is no easily accessible program available, despite good evidence for the efficacy of neuromuscular agility training in the prevention of ACL injury. Recent Australian research has shown that a prevention program, targeted to 12- to 25-year-olds participating in high-risk sports, could prevent 40% of ACL injuries in this group, with significant cost savings to the community [4]. A clear opportunity exists here for orthopaedic surgeons as leaders in health advocacy.

I'm also concerned that other well-intentioned interventions to reduce the risk of re-injury in this group may turn out to be of little benefit or even harmful. I am thinking specifically of lateral extra-articular tenodesis, a procedure largely abandoned before but experiencing resurgence in popularity. It would not be the first time we thought we were smarter than our predecessors and reintroduced an orthopaedic concept that has failed before, only for it to fail again. Just look at metal on metal hip replacements.

So, what happened to my kid? Well, he returned to play 15 months after his reconstruction, having missed a season and a half. In his first game back, he sustained a concussion, missed several more weeks, and then suffered another season ending injury with a hand fracture requiring surgery. Perhaps, I need not worry quite so much about his knee.

References

1. Webster KE, Feller JA, Leigh WB, Richmond AK. Younger patients are at increased risk for graft rupture and contralateral injury after anterior cruciate ligament reconstruction. Am J Sports Med. 2014;42(3):641–7.
2. Zbrojkiewicz D, Vertullo C, Grayson JE. Increasing rates of anterior cruciate ligament reconstruction in young Australians, 2000-2015. Med J Aust. 2018;208(8):354–8.
3. Arendt E, Dick R. Knee injury patterns among men and women in collegiate basketball and soccer. NCAA data and review of literature. Am J Sports Med. 1995;23(6):694–701.
4. Lewis DA, Kirkbride B, Vertullo CJ, Gordon L, Comans TA. Comparison of four alternative national universal anterior cruciate ligament injury prevention programme implementation strategies to reduce secondary future medical costs. Br J Sports Med. 2018;52(4):277–82.

Mentoring in Orthopaedic Sports Medicine

48

Robert F. LaPrade

I believe it is very important that those of us in leadership positions to try and mentor the future generation of young physicians in orthopaedic sports medicine as much as we can. As we have all become busier and the workload of our documentation and paperwork has significantly increased and consumed our time, we are spending less time teaching and laying hands on patients than those physicians of previous generations.

Therefore, one of the important goals that we should set for the future of sports medicine is to ensure that we all spend adequate time in the instruction of our medical students, residents and fellows on the proper listening skills, examination skills and surgical skills to best treat our patients. We can all only teach the younger generation so many things, and by being good teachers, hopefully, this will further expand the knowledge base of all sports medicine physicians and physician extenders as they go on to teach others through our example.

There are many ways that we as orthopaedic leaders can help to mentor young orthopaedic sports surgeons. Some simple ways are to go out of one's way to find residents and fellows when one has an interesting case that is rare. This would give them the opportunity to both see the case and also to be able to ask questions to enhance their knowledge base and ensure that they recognize this pathology if they encounter it in the future. In other words, it is important to ensure that they see it and that it just doesn't see them! Other ways are to encourage residents and fellows to see complex cases in clinic and then to review those cases with them in detail to ensure that their diagnosis is correct and then to explore the intricacies of both the history and physical exam. Other ways are to encourage the residents and fellows attend the examination under anaesthesia of patients with knee ligament pathology, such that their physical examination skills can be enhanced.

R. F. LaPrade (✉)
Twin Cities Orthopedics, Edina, MN, USA

© ISAKOS 2020

123

B. M. Devitt et al. (eds.), *The Future of Orthopaedic Sports Medicine*,
https://doi.org/10.1007/978-3-030-28976-8_48

A further method to engage in mentoring is to involve residents and fellows with research projects. Providing them with true hands-on projects, where they are the first author, helps to encourage them to pursue other projects and to develop a thirst to do further research projects. In my own case, I believe that every project I have ever worked on has enhanced my history and physical examination skills, and being able to encourage our younger generation by mentoring them to learn this and perform it in their own career is important.

Other ways that we can improve our mentorship skills are to place residents and young practicing orthopaedic surgeons on committees. I have found that all the committees for the major sports medicine groups have good niches for encouraging one to interact with other peers and to enhance one's knowledge base in many areas of orthopaedic surgery.

Finally, other important ways of mentoring our younger orthopaedic surgeons and fellows are to be responsible in responding back when they have tough cases. Nowadays, I find that I receive PowerPoint presentations of difficult cases from former fellows and young attendings almost two to three times a week. Taking the time to review these cases thoughtfully; respond back to them with treatment options and also pointing out some of the nuances of the videos, exam or MRI scans within 24–48 h should help them to enhance their ability to take care of complex cases going forward.

Unfortunately, the science of mentoring is not well taught in the medical field. In fact, it is most often instructed by observation. In order to best hand-down our knowledge base and to have the best clinicians in our field going forward, all of us in my generation should strive hard to provide the best examples for teaching, and ultimately mentoring, to the younger generation of sports medicine physicians to ensure that our patients have the best care possible.

Jorge Mineiro

Globalization has produced several standards in Orthopaedics and Traumatology that stand as guidelines for good practice, both in sports medicine and in many other fields. Certification of medical professionals has resulted in a guarantee of quality for the general public, which would otherwise have been difficult to obtain. Each country has developed its own standards, but these are all quite different, at least in Europe, and quite varied. When we examine these standards in detail, they are very closely related to the health care systems around the world, as in each European country.

With the free movement of professionals that was introduced by the Treaty of Rome in 1957, the ability of clinicians began to be judged according to their country of origin and not by their training and competence.

As in the United States, the European Union felt the need to harmonize the different qualifications that existed in order to provide a better service to the public throughout Europe, taking into account that although national qualifications were legally accepted throughout the EU, the truth is that there was no automatic acceptance of specialist qualifications by any institution. Therefore, the need for a Europe-wide specialist qualification became necessary. A qualification that would be issued with the support of the different European orthopaedic societies would have a much wider acceptance by both national societies and regulatory authorities. UEMS (Union of European Medical Specialists), after much discussion, currently favours European qualifications as an alternative to, or in addition to, national ones.

J. Mineiro (✉)
University of Lisbon, Lisbon, Portugal

Hospital Dª Estefania, Lisbon, Portugal

Hospital CUF Descobertas, Lisbon, Portugal
e-mail: jmineiro@netcabo.pt

© ISAKOS 2020
B. M. Devitt et al. (eds.), *The Future of Orthopaedic Sports Medicine*,
https://doi.org/10.1007/978-3-030-28976-8_49

So, although general training in orthopaedics is today regulated nationally, there is an increasing trend for each speciality to have a European board qualification for specialists that will one day replace national qualifications in the whole of Europe.

However, at present, due to the different languages spoken in the EU, the practical side of the Diploma that tests clinical skills, attitude and professional behaviour is still in preparation, due to the fact that some European countries are not prepared to allow their clinicians to go through this process of appraisal! Many different objections are raised: "it is not legal to use patients for medical exams; what if patients require payment to participate in clinical examinations; it will not be possible to conduct examinations in hospitals; etc…"

In my own view, assessment of this step is essential to guarantee that doctors who obtain a specialist qualification know how to examine patients and can make informed decisions regarding management of each of the patient's conditions.

The national orthopaedic societies should be and have been concerned with this level of knowledge and skills amongst their members. When assessing trainees who wish to embark upon specialist practice, examiners are concerned with technical skills, as well as a comprehensive knowledge base. An understanding of the investigation of patients with complex problems, leading to correct decisions regarding management is also required, to improve the patient's condition. This level of expert training and assessment is usually carried out after general training in orthopaedics and should be under the guidance of the Speciality Societies of Europe. They should provide not only training centres but also diplomas, which are beyond the competence of general orthopaedic departments. Specialist training in different areas is usually undertaken as fellowships and is provided by recognized centres that fulfil certain criteria. On completion of such a fellowship, with a European general qualification and a specialist diploma, the clinician should be able to deal with the more complex pathologies. As far as the public is concerned, such a clinician is a certified specialist able to solve their problem.

Although this is the correct flowchart for specialist training in the Western world, other views regarding specialised training have been raised—should such doctors be the only ones fully licensed to manage the more and the less complex pathology of an anatomic area? Do we have enough of these specialists to cover all health care systems? If not, we are in a very grey area regarding responsibility—if there are not enough super specialists to cover all hospitals, how can we structure the rules for referral? To what extent is the fully qualified competent general orthopaedic surgeon in Europe able to look after specific conditions in a general hospital? We see in many countries in Europe patients being referred great distances because doctors on the premises are not 'licensed' to do a particular operation, and this can be applied to the different areas in the field of trauma or orthopaedics: from a common Colles fracture, carpal tunnel syndrome, bunion, torn meniscus, fractured tibial plateau fracture of the proximal humerus, herniated lumbar disc, etc.…

We have all faced similar dilemmas through life! In a hostile environment, through pressure from lawyers, administrators and sport managers, it is often difficult to distinguish what is a recognised complication of a complex condition from a technical mistake or even negligent practice. It can also be difficult to judge when is the right time to allow patients to resume their physical activities in sports or other professional activities when their condition is still not fully recovered. The effectiveness of particular procedures, especially regarding recovery time and its financial implications, now play a major role in clinical management. How do we draw the line between the tasks of the generalist and the super-specialist?

Regarding certification, which is the best option—to know how to examine a patient, value his/her symptoms and physical signs and use that information to help make an informed decision regarding treatment or to be a super skilful technician able to perform the most complex procedure, given an established diagnosis? At the present time, these two scenarios do exist, but the articulation between them is not optimized due to lack of scientific rigour in establishing outcomes—in other words, evidence-based medicine.

The task for both national and speciality societies in Europe is enormous, trying to make sure these two types of orthopaedists are fully trained and that the super-specialist will never be able to get to this level of competence without completing successfully general training in the speciality—it is fantastic to have a skilled surgeon doing a difficult total knee replacement (TKR), but he/she also needs to be able to recognize a post-operative compartment syndrome! On the other hand, it is the responsibility of the Head of Training to make sure that residents get appropriate general training and do not go into specialized training too early. It is the task of the European Board examiners to make sure that general knowledge in orthopaedics and trauma is covered in the appraisal at the end of orthopaedic and trauma residency. Technical details about less common procedures should be left for the assessment at the end of specific fellowships and therefore for a different setup.

Awareness of these issues will, I am confident, bring solutions for training, which will ensure better care of all patients with musculoskeletal disease or injury.

Technology and Sports Medicine: The Good, the Bad and the Ugly

Moisés Cohen

The breakthroughs that technology has provided to medicine, in particular to the orthopaedic sports medicine field, in the past decades are fascinating. At the same time, the advances are progressing so rapidly and exponentially that they can be sometimes overwhelming and, just like in any other area, may also have drawbacks or even potentially be used for questionable purposes.

50.1 The Good

I remember the days when radiographs were our only resource to have a look inside our patients' bodies and to assist us in the decision-making process together with physical examination; that was—and should still be—our most powerful resource. Following this, computed tomography and, more importantly, magnetic resonance imaging (MRI) were introduced into our daily practice, improving remarkably our understanding of the changes taking place in our patients, in a non-invasive manner. Technology also significantly improved our ability to treat injuries that were once career-ending to many athletes in the past. Nowadays, patients with threatening injuries such as with knee dislocations and multiple ligaments injuries have successfully returned to sport. The advent of arthroscopy and the constant evolution of materials and techniques to perform less invasive surgeries have also been playing a critical role to help us improve patient care.

M. Cohen (✉)
Department of Orthopaedics and Traumatology, Federal University of São Paulo, São Paulo, Brazil

© ISAKOS 2020
B. M. Devitt et al. (eds.), *The Future of Orthopaedic Sports Medicine*,
https://doi.org/10.1007/978-3-030-28976-8_50

50.2   The Bad

Technology is everywhere and is playing an increasing role in our clinical setting. It is common to see in current practice a patient with a straightforward complaint undergoing multiple investigative examinations, which are of dubious benefit. Worse still, unfortunately and not infrequently, treatments are based solely on the imaging findings rather than on the patient's complaints, with less time being invested in a thorough physical examination. I believe we must be conscious about not only the benefits but also the limitations of the technological advancements in our practice; it can support us to provide optimal patient care, although we must not forget that medical care should still be centred around the patient's complaints and physical examination.

50.3   The Ugly

The technology advancements, more specifically in the field of genetics, are very promising for the treatment of diseases related to the expression or lack of expression of genes. However, this gene therapy field can theoretically be also used for other purposes, such as enhancement of athletic performance, or so-called 'gene doping'. Since the discovery in the last decade that the insertion of a gene into muscle cells in rats leads to cell growth, the use of genes to improve athletes' physical abilities has become a reality. In time, they will most likely take the place of the current illegal substances that are strictly prohibited in competitive and professional sports. The issue is this new raft of 'cheating' may potentially be undiscoverable, go uncontrolled and have drastic long-term consequences. This could lead to a total shift in competitive sports. It could possibly transform into a competition between which team or player has the best genetic engineering technology, and not between talent and hard work.

Therefore, I believe that we must keep our minds open for the improvements and benefits that technology can provide us in our practice in the orthopaedic sports medicine field but also have a critical view of the use of new high-tech tools for clinical practice and sports.

Will It Be Possible to Perform a 99%
Perfect ACL Reconstruction
in the Future?

51

Joon Ho Wang

As a result of advances in surgical techniques, clinical results after surgical treatment for anterior cruciate ligament (ACL) reconstruction have improved greatly. However, there are still a lot of unsatisfactory outcomes. Many doctors agree that problems still exist with current surgical techniques and treatment strategies. We believe further improvements in surgical methods are yet to be devised. In order to better understand the future of ACL surgery, we must know more about current surgical procedures and their issues.

For ACL reconstruction using an autograft, the graft is prepared by harvesting tendons. Whilst allografts are available for ACL reconstruction, supply could be limited depending on global location and time. The harvested tendon is usually prepared in a simple cylindrical shaped graft, which differs from the bow-tie shape of the original ACL, which is narrow at the middle and broader region of the femoral and tibial attachment sites. It is also difficult to mimic the enthesis of the ACL on the bone. Instead of attaching the graft to the bony surface, the graft is passed through an artificially drilled femoral and tibial tunnel at the anatomic insertion site and fixed with the graft. The implanted ligament should heal on the bone. After revascularization in the ligamentization process, vascularity of the graft might not be as much as a normal ACL. Its strength is usually weaker than that of a normal ACL, which leaves it susceptible to further tearing even by a minor trauma. One solution to these issues could be to make artificial grafts by tissue-engineered methods, including 3D bio-printing technology. A tissue-engineered ACL graft with a bow-tie appearance, rather than a cylindrical one, could be produced by printing stem cells, fibroblast, and angioblast with a scaffold such as collagen gel and polycaprolactic acid. Dual printing technology, which involves printing stem cells and scaffold by using dual printing nodules, could make it possible to print

J. H. Wang (✉)
Department of Orthopedic Surgery, Samsung Medical Center, Seoul, Republic of Korea

Department of Orthopedic Surgery, Sungkyunkwan University School of Medicine, Seoul, Republic of Korea

© ISAKOS 2020
B. M. Devitt et al. (eds.), *The Future of Orthopaedic Sports Medicine*,
https://doi.org/10.1007/978-3-030-28976-8_51

3D structured grafts with stem cells. Alternatively, electro-spinning technology could be used for the fabrication of ACL using nano- or micro-fibers from silk material or other polymers. It might also be possible to achieve a strong attachment of graft to bone without the need for drilling, by using a bone-tendon complex graft, made with 3D printing technology, which could print both the bony and ligament parts of the graft continuously.

For successful ligamentization, in-growth of blood vessels into the graft is necessary. By attaching the VGEF to the surface of tissue-engineered graft fibers, revascularization of the graft could be promoted. By promoting the re-growth of new blood vessels, we could expect faster ligamentization due to promoted migration of fibroblast resulting in an increased survival rate of the graft. The regenerated ligaments could produce enough collagen to be as strong as a normal ACL. Whilst we can't be sure all issues regarding ACL grafts can be solved by using 3D printing technology, technical hurdles are being removed one by one by many researchers and clinicians. By improving the techniques involved in image analyzing research, we could eventually make customized tissue-engineered grafts, which exactly match patients' original ligament shape.

Is it possible to perform 99% perfect ACL reconstruction using new technology?

Yes it is. But right now, it is difficult to say exactly when that will be achieved.

The Good and the Bad of Evidence-Based Medicine and the Challenge of Practising in a Time of Increased Connectivity and Artificial Intelligence

52

David A. Parker

As we move well into the twenty-first century, the concept of evidence-based medicine is well established, and surgeons will become more obliged to practise medicine along these lines. Of course they should, we hear commentators say, and it certainly does make sense to have evidence for what we do when we choose to operate on people. The difficulty is deciding on what level of evidence is sufficient—at one extreme, we may think that knowing that something has 'worked well in our hands' should be enough to justify what we do, whereas at the other extreme, randomized controlled trials (RCT) or meta-analyses thereof may be considered by some as required to really have sufficient evidence. We all know the flaws of the first extreme, having been taught well by history and proper follow-up that our intuition isn't always right, but the second extreme also has flaws, in that many conditions aren't suited to RCTs and even with those that are, statistical methods averaging out results will tend to miss those "outsiders" who may have benefited from surgery when the average result found that surgery was not beneficial. We all know that those paying for surgery—government bodies and private health funds—are constantly looking for ways to reduce costs and declining to pay for procedures with insufficient 'evidence' is one way they will always be looking at to achieve this. We are already seeing the impact this is having on arthroscopic knee surgery, not long ago the most common orthopaedic sports medicine procedure performed. It won't be enough for surgeons to expect funding for a procedure just because they believe it is right, and surgeons will need to be proactive and take the lead in providing the necessary evidence by studying carefully and scientifically what they do. Once funding is removed from a procedure, it will be very hard to get it back.

Increased connectivity of the world through social media, and the development of artificial intelligence (AI) will also create a completely different environment in which we will be practising surgery and other areas of medicine. Increased levels of

D. A. Parker (✉)
Sydney Orthopaedic Research Institute, Sydney, NSW, Australia
e-mail: dparker@sydneyortho.com.au

© ISAKOS 2020
B. M. Devitt et al. (eds.), *The Future of Orthopaedic Sports Medicine*,
https://doi.org/10.1007/978-3-030-28976-8_52

promotion of surgeons and techniques, by surgeons themselves and industry, will create pressure on surgeons to 'advertise or die' and also adhere to more popular and easily promoted techniques that attract more business, very much in the way politicians have populist policies to garner more votes. We are already seeing these pressures existing for some time in countries like the USA, and gradually creeping into other countries, making it difficult for doctors to not lose sight of the basic principle of medicine, which is to always give advice and provide treatment primarily in the patient's interest. The increased development of artificial intelligence is already greatly influencing the way we live our lives, and is already having an impact on medicine. AI has already been shown to be more accurate in some imaging interpretation in radiology than humans, and there is no doubt that anything with a predictable pattern or algorithm that can be automated will be, and doctors will be beholden to provide evidence, as outlined in the above paragraph, that the 'human factor' is actually better if it is to persist. Most importantly, doctors need to embrace rather than shun and vilify this technology. We will only remain in the position of power in patient management if we control the technology that is used for it.

Preventing Osteoarthritis in Young Patients After Anterior Cruciate Ligament Injury

53

Anastasios Georgoulis

The treatment of the anterior cruciate ligament (ACL)-injured knee has been an exciting challenge, and it will continue to be so for a long time to come. Despite the improvements in our reconstruction techniques, advances in augmented tissue healing, and expansion of our knowledge of the anatomy and biomechanical role of the ACL, there are many questions yet to be answered. And, there is still plenty of room for improvement!

In the short term, there are many reconstruction techniques that can be undertaken to produce a stable knee joint, enabling return to active sports participation following appropriate rehabilitation with physiotherapy and allowing sufficient time for graft healing. However, in the long term, with the goal of preventing osteoarthritis, there is certainly more to do.

The ACL is the guide for internal and external rotation of the knee. During flexion and extension, the knee joint rotates in a synchronized and coordinated manner with the movement of the hip and ankle joints, which are moving above and below, respectively. In the ACL-injured knee, this harmonic movement is disrupted, the center of the rotation of the knee is displaced more medially and posteriorly, resulting in interference in the smooth and coordinated rolling and gliding of the lateral condyle. The consequence of this altered biomechanics, along with the further disorder that chondral and meniscal injury causes, results in the development of osteoarthritis in the medium to long term.

To achieve the requisite stability of the knee joint to enables return to sports participation and prevention the development of osteoarthritis, it is felt that an anatomical ACL reconstruction is needed.

This term was coined by my mentor, Peter Hertel, who taught me arthroscopy and ACL reconstruction surgery. The phrase was first used by him at the ESSKA

A. Georgoulis (✉)
Orthopaedic Surgery Department, Hygeia and Metropolitan Hospital, Athens, Greece

University Hospital of Ioannina, Ioannina, Greece

© ISAKOS 2020

B. M. Devitt et al. (eds.), *The Future of Orthopaedic Sports Medicine*,
https://doi.org/10.1007/978-3-030-28976-8_53

congress in Stockholm in 1990 when he proposed a "patellar tendon graft" placed in the anatomic insertions of the native ACL. Biomechanical laboratory studies of our own along with others underlined the necessity to correct not only the anterior tibial translation but also the pathological rotation to re-establish normal knee kinematics.

Freddie Fu introduced the idea of the anatomic reconstruction using the double bundle technique to manage both problems. It was suggested that both bundles could achieve the short-term goal of stabilization of the knee but also restore abnormal rotation and prevention of osteoarthritis as well. His enthusiasm and the seminal research he produced was the initiation for new discussion. Japan, with its leaders K. Shino, M. Ochi, H. Kurosaka, K. Yasuda, and others, contributed substantially to the better understanding of the anatomy and biomechanics of the ACL-injured and reconstructed knee. In addition, G. Cerulli introduced the concept of a minimally invasive technique, using only a single hamstring, to reconstruction of the ACL with short tunnels.

If we consider that this operation determines if a young person will continue to be active for his/her entire life, we can understand that this procedure is not so simple. We have to use a graft that is, although similar to the native ACL, is not quite the same. Perhaps, in the near future, we will be able to produce a graft using stem cells from the patient themselves.

The surgeon has to be able to place the femoral tunnel in anatomic position using the antero-medial or the lateral approach and not the transtibial one, in order that the graft has a similar obliquity as that of the native ACL. During fixation, the subluxation of the knee has to be diminished, and the preinjury orientation of the PCL needs to be corrected. Only in this way, can we reconstruct the ACL anatomically giving long-term stability and avoiding osteoarthritis. Otherwise, we will have a large number of re-ruptures and the development of early osteoarthritis in young patients. My fear is that poor surgery and the resultant suboptimal results give this procedure a bad name. It provides ammunition for those against the idea of surgery to justify their claims. Intensive education on the correct technique and further research will lead to more and more successful results following treatment of ACL injuries.

The Danger of Making Decisions for Evolution, Quality of Care, and Education Based on National Health Data

54

Björn Barenius

Swedish healthcare often gets praise for its quality and effectiveness. With our individual PIN number, all Swedish National's visits in the health system can be followed. In Sweden, there is a strong dominance for tax-financed healthcare. We Swedes in general feel secure that the social system protects our interests. The quality and effectiveness of the healthcare provided in the different regions are regulated and assessed by the Swedish National Board of Health and Welfare and the Swedish Association of Local Authorities and Regions. The Swedish Association of Local Authorities and Regions have published international comparisons since 2005. In these publications, Sweden is often among the top countries in the world according to the assessed indexes. The Swedish prosthesis registries and the knee ligament register are world famous for their detailed data on subjective and objective results at a national level. So, what is there to worry about?

As an orthopedic sport medicine surgeon, I worry that the Swedish healthcare system is too focused on effectivity and being cost-oriented to have room for education and evolution of new treatment options. In my mind, the reports above have led the organizations regulating the health care system to base their decisions on the economy and not on quality (because quality as assessed in the reports is always top notch). The regulators are only concerned with effectiveness and the cost of the produced healthcare. One of the latest projects in healthcare regulation is to export routine care from hospitals to private units. Hospital care is expensive, and private units are more cost-efficient. Compensation is determined according to a predetermined pricelist, which is based on diagnosis and not on the performed procedure, need for a particular implant, or the performed surgeon-to-surgeon education. Consequently, in a country where surgeons are starved of private opportunities, a number of actors have emerged. A small private unit with one or a few experienced surgeons working fast on their own with a minimalistic approach to implants can get

B. Barenius (✉)
Department of Clinical Science and Education, Södersjukhuset,
Karolinska Institutet, Stockholm, Sweden

© ISAKOS 2020
B. M. Devitt et al. (eds.), *The Future of Orthopaedic Sports Medicine*,
https://doi.org/10.1007/978-3-030-28976-8_54

enough money to become financially independent. Sports medicine is mostly composed of healthy individuals with traumatic injuries, that is, well suited for the private unit. *"But this type of system has worked for us"* you might reply if you're coming from the US or a number of European countries. Why can't you make it work in Sweden?

In time, we might raise the awareness of quality and education in the private sector as well as in hospital units. However, a Swedish surgical residency is based on working at a hospital for 5–6 years. During that time, new techniques and the honing of clinical and surgical skills are taught through a system of apprenticeship. The system of fellowship training is nonexistent in Sweden. After residency, it is common to stay at the same hospital focusing on a sub-specialty with continued surgeon-to-surgeon learning. Many residents in university hospitals have had time to reflect on clinical problems and might have found a special area of interest, maybe embarking on a PhD education, to get into their preferred sub-specialty field.

I worry that the new project in healthcare regulation has not allotted funds for education or research outside the public hospitals. From a shortsighted national economic perspective, it might save money to treat only the very sick or in need of advanced costly care in the university hospitals and the routine cases in the private sector. However, with this division, the early resident's educational need with routine cases is lost, and so is the future patients' need for surgeons trained in all surgical techniques.

If all arthroscopic surgeries are performed in a setting without apprenticeship and under hard productive pressure: Who will transfer the knowledge of sports medicine surgery? Who will secure that the quality of care is maintained? And who will find time to evolve new methods and perform the studies needed to test them?

When Dogmas Are Not Revised Soon, Our Sportsmen's Hips and Knees Will Not Be Preserved but Instead Replaced

55

Ronald van Heerwaarden

Dogmas, defined as principles or sets of principles laid down by an authority as the incontrovertible truth, are widespread in use in medicine. Described in textbooks and taught by our teachers, they represent the backbone of our knowledge and are often the basis of our everyday practice.

The problem with dogmas is that they may represent old knowledge based on sometimes little scientific proof and expert opinions. At the time the dogmas evolved, however, for the authority or authorities, it may as well have been the only available knowledge and therewith conceived as the undisputed truth. Whereas some dogmas, first stated many decades ago, may still hold the undisputable truth, other dogmas are considered old, as, in the meantime, the principles have been proven wrong or are replaced by a new dogma laid down by a new authority. Examples of old dogmas described in the field of orthopaedics and sports medicine are that the best way to treat a meniscus tear is to perform a total meniscectomy, chondroplasty is the best way to treat cartilage damage and that joint replacements are indicated for the elderly that lead a sedentary life.

Teaching our young doctors can be compared to unfolding an old map representing the world of medical knowledge. On this map, the main roads are paved with stones of scientifically proven knowledge and undisputable dogmas. History has thought us where the main roads are for the best treatments of our patients based on the highest levels of knowledge. Teaching also includes preventing our young colleagues not to get side-tracked off the main road. We can do this by pointing out that besides the main roads, old and new paths exist paved with old dogmas and unproven concepts. Lessons have been learned from old dogmas proven wrong and premature adoption of knowledge without sound scientific proof.

History, however, has not taught us enough lessons yet. Already decades ago, metal-metal hip prostheses were considered on a side-track after abundant scientific

R. van Heerwaarden (✉)
Centre for Deformity Correction and Joint Preserving Surgery, Kliniek ViaSana, Mill, The Netherlands

© ISAKOS 2020
B. M. Devitt et al. (eds.), *The Future of Orthopaedic Sports Medicine*,
https://doi.org/10.1007/978-3-030-28976-8_55

139

proof of failures. However, in recent years, a new dogma was created for the treatment of the young patient with hip osteoarthritis, the so-called 'sports hip', an improved metal-metal hip prosthesis. After the re-birth of the metal-metal implant, the demise of the new dogma was clear after only a few years as scientific proof of unacceptable failure rates became apparent. Time will tell whether current days' joint replacement treatments advertised for younger patients will end along the same road in early revisions.

On the main road of orthopaedics, a dogma can be found stating that joint replacements have been proven to be one of the best orthopaedic procedures for elderly patients with severe osteoarthritis leading a sedentary life. A huge and ever-increasing amount of scientific proof supports this dogma; however, it is dangerous to use this scientific proof to pave new roads for new dogmas. In the past decades, exits to new roads have been created for the use of joint replacements in younger patients with less severe degrees of osteoarthritis and a new dogma was born that this treatment would be equally effective in younger age. The alarmingly high number of hip and knee replacements performed worldwide in patients under 55 years old shows that we have been side-tracked and, not surprisingly, the scientific proof of increased failure rates in growing rapidly. Further down that road, we see a staggering revision rate of these joint prostheses performed in middle-aged patients that will have an uncertain future, as no knowledge is available of survival of revision hip and knee replacements implanted in this age cohort.

The question is how to keep our young doctors on the main road and preserve our young patients' precious joints instead of replacing them. Only if old dogmas will be systematically revised by evidence-based evaluation tools that nowadays are widely available, new common knowledge will grow and replace the old knowledge. Then new rules should prevent us from creating new roads as side-tracks of the main road.

Christopher D. Harner

In the interest of full disclosure, I am a past American Orthopaedic Society for Sports Medicine (AOSSM) Traveling Fellow (1990 to Europe), a recent Godfather for the AOSSM Traveling Fellowship (2018 to Europe). I have been a member of ISAKOS since 1987 [this was pre-ISAKOS and known as the International Arthroscopy Association (IAA) and International Society of the Knee (ISK)]. I have attended most of the ISAKOS meetings over the past 30 years, I have served on the Program Committee, Executive Committee and Board of Directors and I love this organization.

Since I am a positive person, I would like to change the focus of this narrative from 'What Should We Be Worried About?' to 'What Should We Be Excited About?' I believe that the key to our future of orthopedic sports medicine is to remain as a sub-specialty of orthopedic surgery and not be confused with other non-surgical sports medicine groups (primary care sports medicine, athletic training, physical therapy, etc.). We are orthopedic surgeons whose strength is understanding the art and science of musculoskeletal care in active individuals from pediatrics to geriatrics. We are skilled in the art and science of non-operative and operative management in active individuals (recreational to professional) of all ages.

Our commitment to a scientific body of knowledge (orthopedic sports medicine) with research and education to back up our treatments is critical. This responsibility does not come easily and must be continuously and relentlessly pursued by setting the intellectual and educational bar as high as possible. Lifelong learning for us is a mission and not a mandate. ISAKOS remains a critical organization for us to achieve this mission through continuing medical education. We pride ourselves in being the organization for international collaboration of orthopedic leaders whose focus is education and research with a particular emphasis on honesty and intellectual

C. D. Harner (✉)
Department of Orthopaedics, University of Texas McGovern Medical School,
Houston, TX, USA
e-mail: christopher.harner@uth.tmc.edu

© ISAKOS 2020 141
B. M. Devitt et al. (eds.), *The Future of Orthopaedic Sports Medicine*,
https://doi.org/10.1007/978-3-030-28976-8_56

integrity. We have had the great fortune to have an Executive Director, Michele Johnson, with us for the majority of our existence. Now that Michele will be stepping down, our next challenge will be to maintain and strengthen our mission to be the world leader in orthopedic sports medicine. I am confident with our current and future international leadership that we will continue to maintain and strengthen our mission to advance the worldwide exchange and dissemination of education, research, and patient care in arthroscopy, knee surgery and orthopaedic sports medicine.

A Lot Done, More to Do!

57

João Espregueira-Mendes

Nowadays, we have a very active population. In particular, we have seen an increase in recent times in the activity levels of children and elderly; not only are numbers of participants in sport increasing in these age groups, but they are also engaging in sports at higher intensity than previously seen in previous generations. This phenomenon is responsible for the appearance of specific lesions that were unusual in these age groups heretofore.

The state-of-art treatment of patients with an open physis has changed over the years. Previously, we adopted a predominantly non-operative approach, but we are increasingly aware of the potentially harmful consequences of postponing surgical treatments in many of these patients, particularly those presenting with ligament, cartilage, and meniscal injuries. As such, these lesions are now more frequently treated surgically. However, the outcomes must be improved, especially when considering that there are still potential side effects that we cannot fully understand and explain.

The older age group represents an even more demanding group of patients. These are nowadays much more active and whose expectations of surgery are not just mere pain relief but improved function and restoration of normal activity. The re-establishment of function and sport capabilities for elderly patients is another worrisome concern for the future. Joint degenerative diseases affect a considerable proportion of this group of patients and this number will increase in future with the increase in life expectancy of our population. As it stands, our gold standard procedures for the

J. Espregueira-Mendes (✉)
Clínica do Dragão, Espregueira-Mendes Sports Centre—FIFA Medical Centre of Excellence, Porto, Portugal

Dom Henrique Research Centre, Porto, Portugal

ICVS/3B's, PT Government Associated Laboratory, Braga/Guimarães, Portugal

School of Medicine, Minho University, Braga, Portugal
e-mail: jem@espregueira.com

© ISAKOS 2020
B. M. Devitt et al. (eds.), *The Future of Orthopaedic Sports Medicine*,
https://doi.org/10.1007/978-3-030-28976-8_57

treatment of severe joint degeneration with joint arthroplasties are incapable of meeting the expectation of this patient group. Perhaps, biologic injectable therapies will provide the answer in the future?

For those patients that lie between these two age spectrums, anterior cruciate ligament (ACL) rupture is a severe injury that many athletes face during their sporting careers. As we know, this injury results in a long layoff period and extensive rehabilitation. Although a reasonable percentage of athletes return to sport, many of them do not return to their pre-injury level of competition, and we still face an unacceptable high reinjury rate. Moreover, even when we consider a reconstruction is 'successful', we still are unable to restore normal knee kinematics and prevent the development of early osteoarthritis. We must better understand the influence of morphologic knee factors in the joint stability and their role in treatment outcomes. There are several other questions that we also need to answer: Why do we see patients with isolated total ACL lesions with explosive lateral pivot shift and others with the same lesion with a very small rotation laxity? Why do we have partial lesions with an explosive lateral pivot shift? How can we be sure that a remaining bundle in a partial ACL rupture is functioning and how can we correctly measure laxity in this context?

Meniscal lesions are also a common knee injury, in particular, in the middle-age active population. The importance of preservation of meniscal tissue must be a concern for the future. Meniscal repair has been regarded as a beneficial technique for preserving meniscal tissue. Meniscal allograft transplantation and meniscal scaffold substitution are also available options. However, these do not guarantee a complete return to sport and often result in a prolonged layoff also with extensive rehabilitation. In addition, not all athletes with meniscal injuries are candidates for meniscal repair or substitution, and the protracted rehabilitation period often makes repair or restorative procedures a non-viable option for competing athletes. Thus, partial or total meniscectomy is more often considered, which, although providing a high rate and fast return to sports, is associated with sub-optimal long-term outcomes and the early development of knee osteoarthritis. Meniscal repair equipment is expensive and not always available in many cases for surgeons and patients due to economic constraints. There is also an issue with training of surgeons to perform meniscal repair. This is not only related to the cost of the procedure and therefore the lack of exposure of trainees to this technique in the public sector but also the lack of availability to educational programmes, which needs improvement. There is still an important gap between evidence and clinical practice in terms of meniscal surgery. The role of meniscectomies has to be re-evaluated, and a consensus about the treatment of meniscal lesions must be discussed. We still do not know how much meniscus we can remove without changing the biomechanics and causing osteoarthritis. How much is too much?

Another frequent problem found in orthopaedic sports medicine is damage to articular cartilage. We do not know why some cartilage lesions give pain and others do not, and why do we have pain free periods in the same cartilage lesion? Many advanced cartilage restoration techniques have emerged, and despite our great efforts in applying and refining these techniques, the results are not sufficient and we are still not able to restore normal hyaline cartilage. For the future, we should be worried about not only providing pain relief and improvement of quality of life for our patients but also re-establishing a high level of sport activity. Tissue engineering and novel technologies of reparative medicine have a fundamental role in this particular field and may be the future.

We have achieved outstanding improvements in managing orthopaedic sports injuries, but we still need to keep improving and re-invent ourselves to provide our patients with the best possible solution.